SOMNOLOGY Jr. 2
Pocket Sleep Medicine

Teofilo Lee-Chiong MD
Somnologist

To Grace Zamudio and Zoe Lee-Chiong

Teofilo Lee-Chiong MD

Chief Medical Liaison
Philips Respironics

Professor of Medicine
National Jewish Health
Denver, Colorado

Professor of Medicine
University of Colorado Denver
School of Medicine
Aurora, Colorado

Preface to the second edition
Dormitatis ergo estis.

Preface to the first edition
Carpe noctem.

Abbreviations

ABG	Arterial blood gas
AC	Alternating current
ACTH	Adrenocorticotropic hormone
ADH	Antidiuretic hormone
ADHD	Attention deficit hyperactivity disorder
AF	Atrial fibrillation
AHI	Apnea hypopnea index
AI	Apnea index
ALTE	Apparent life-threatening event
ANS	Autonomic nervous system
APAP	Auto-titrating positive airway pressure
ASPS	Advanced sleep phase syndrome
ASV	Adaptive servo ventilation
AVAPS	Average volume assured pressure support
BMI	Body mass index
BP	Blood pressure
BPAP	Bi-level positive airway pressure
BZ	Benzodiazepine
CA	Central apnea
CAD	Coronary artery disease
CBT-I	Cognitive behavioral therapy for insomnia
CFlex	CPAP with expiratory pressure relief
CHF	Congestive heart failure
CNS	Central nervous system
CO	Cardiac output
CO_2	Carbon dioxide
COPD	Chronic obstructive pulmonary disease
CPAP	Continuous positive airway pressure
CRSD	Circadian rhythm sleep disorder
CRP	C-reactive protein
CSA	Central sleep apnea
CSF	Cerebrospinal fluid
CSR	Cheyne Stokes respiration
CT	Computed tomography
CTmin	Minimum core body temperature
DC	Direct current
DLMO	Dim light melatonin onset
DM	Diabetes mellitus
DSPS	Delayed sleep phase syndrome
DZ	Dizygotic
ECG	Electrocardiography
EDS	Excessive daytime sleepiness

EEG	Electroencephalography	IL	Interleukin
EMG	Electromyography	IPAP	Inspiratory positive airway pressure
EOG	Electro-oculography	ISWR	Irregular sleep-wake rhythm
EPAP	Expiratory positive airway pressure	JL	Jet lag
ESRD	End-stage renal disease	LDT	Laterodorsal tegmentum
ESS	Epworth sleepiness scale	LV	Left ventricle
FDA	Food and Drug Administration	LVEF	Left ventricular ejection fraction
FEV_1	Forced expiratory volume in 1 second	MAOI	Monoamine oxidase inhibitor
FRD	Free running disorder	MRI	Magnetic resonance imaging
FVC	Forced vital capacity	MSLT	Multiple sleep latency test
GABA	Gamma-aminobutyric acid	MWT	Maintenance of wakefulness test
GER	Gastroesophageal reflux	MZ	Monozygotic
GFR	Glomerular filtration rate	N1	NREM stage 1 sleep
GH	Growth hormone	N2	NREM stage 2 sleep
GHB	Gamma hydroxybutyrate	N3	NREM stages 3 (and 4) sleep
Hcrt	Hypocretin	NBBRA	Non-benzodiazepine benzodiazepine receptor agonist
HIV	Human immunodeficiency virus	NIPPV	Non-invasive positive pressure ventilation
HLA	Human leukocyte antigen	NREM	Non-rapid eye movement sleep
HR	Heart rate	O_2	Oxygen
HTN	Hypertension	ODI	Oxygen desaturation index
Hz	Hertz (cycles per second)		

OHS	Obesity hypoventilation syndrome	R	Stage REM sleep
OSA	Obstructive sleep apnea	RBD	REM sleep behavior disorder
$PaCO_2$	Partial pressure of arterial carbon dioxide	RDI	Respiratory disturbance index
PaO_2	Partial pressure of arterial oxygen	REM	Rapid eye movement sleep
PAP	Positive airway pressure	REM SL	Rapid eye movement sleep latency
PD	Parkinson disease	RIP	Respiratory inductance plethysmography
$PetCO_2$	Partial pressure of end-tidal carbon dioxide	RLS	Restless legs syndrome
PLMD	Periodic limb movement disorder	RR	Respiratory rate
PLMI	Periodic limb movement index	RV	Right ventricle
PLMS	Periodic limb movements of sleep	SaO_2	Oxygen saturation
PLMW	Periodic limb movements of wakefulness	SCN	Suprachiasmatic nucleus
PPT	Pedunculopontine tegmentum	SD	Sleep deprivation
PSAT	Portable sleep apnea testing	SE	Sleep efficiency
PSG	Polysomnography	SNRI	Serotonin and norepinephrine reuptake inhibitor
$PtcCO_2$	Partial pressure of transcutaneous carbon dioxide	SOL	Sleep onset latency
PTSD	Post-traumatic stress disorder	SOREMP	Sleep onset REM period
PUD	Peptic ulcer disease	SRBD	Sleep-related breathing disorder
PVC	Premature ventricular contraction	SSRI	Selective serotonin reuptake inhibitor
PVR	Pulmonary vascular resistance	SVR	Systemic vascular resistance
QOL	Quality of life	SWD	Shift work disorder.

TCA	Tricyclic antidepressant
TIB	Time in bed
TNF	Tumor necrosis factor
TSH	Thyroid stimulating hormone
TST	Total sleep time
TV	Tidal volume
UA	Upper airway
UARS	Upper airway resistance syndrome
VLPO	Ventrolateral preoptic
V/Q	Ventilation-perfusion
W	Stage Wake
WASO	Wake time after sleep onset

Contents

Sleep: a very short introduction

Sleep is a complex reversible state of being. Its principal characteristics include: (a) behavioral quiescence and diminished responsiveness to external stimuli compared to the waking state; (b) stereotypic posture; and (c) rapid state reversibility. Sleep is generated and maintained by central neural networks utilizing specific neurotransmitters that are located in specific areas of the brain. Although a comprehensive theory of the function/s of sleep remains elusive (i.e., sleep may address multiple physiologic needs), it is unquestioned that sleep is central to the development and optimal operation of the brain - neural growth, processing and maturation, neuronal synaptic plasticity, learning, and memory consolidation. Other functions of sleep include restoration and somatic growth, regulation of body temperature, energy conservation, removal of metabolic "toxins" generated during wakefulness, protective and adaptive behavior, and immune defense.

Sleep and wake neurotransmitters

Sleep and wake states are determined by the interaction between wake- and sleep-promoting neurotransmitters. Listed are wake and sleep neurotransmitters and location of their respective neurons.

Wake neurotransmitters	Sleep neurotransmitters
Acetylcholine	Acetylcholine (REM sleep)
Dopamine	Adenosine
Glutamate	GABA
Histamine	Galanin
Hypocretin (orexin)	Glycine
Norepinephrine	Melatonin
Serotonin	

Neurotransmitters	Main location of neurons
Acetylcholine	PPT/LDT and basal forebrain
Adenosine	Basal forebrain
Dopamine	Substantia nigra
GABA	VLPO
Glutamate	Reticular formation, lateral hypothalamus and thalamus
Glycine	Spinal cord
Histamine	Tuberomammillary nucleus
Hypocretin	Hypothalamus (perifornical)
Norepinephrine	Locus coeruleus
Serotonin	Raphe nuclei

Actions of neurotransmitters

Activity of aminergic neurons increases during wake but decreases during NREM and REM sleep. In contrast, activity of cholinergic neurons increases during wake and REM sleep but decreases during NREM sleep.

	Actions
Acetylcholine	Wake and REM sleep neurotransmitter. Responsible for cortical EEG desynchronization during wake and REM sleep.
Adenosine	Sleep neurotransmitter. Responsible for the homeostatic sleep drive. Levels progressively increase during sustained wakefulness and decrease during sustained sleep.
Dopamine	Wake and REM sleep neurotransmitter.
Gamma-aminobutyric acid	Main NREM neurotransmitter. Main CNS inhibitory neurotransmitter.
Glutamate	Main CNS excitatory neurotransmitter. Active during wake and REM sleep.
Glycine	Main inhibitory neurotransmitter in the spinal cord. Responsible for hyperpolarization (inhibition) of spinal motoneurons that causes REM sleep-related muscle atonia/hypotonia.
Histamine	Wake neurotransmitter.
Hypocretin (orexin)	Wake neurotransmitter. Promotes wake and suppresses REM sleep. Acts on other CNS centers related to wake regulation.

Immunomodulators and peptides	IL-Iβ, IL-6, TNFα, prostaglandin D2, delta sleep-inducing peptide, vasoactive intestinal peptide, growth hormone releasing hormone and CRP promote NREM sleep.
Melatonin	Produced by the pineal gland during the biological night. Secretion is inhibited by light exposure. Melatonin receptors are present in the SCN (circadian rhythm regulation) and hypothalamus (thermoregulation).
Norepinephrine	Wake neurotransmitter. Activity of neurons: wake > NREM > REM.
Serotonin	Wake neurotransmitter. Activity of neurons: wake > NREM > REM. Maintains cortical desynchrony during wakefulness.

Sleep and wake neural systems

Wake, NREM sleep and REM sleep are each generated and maintained by different neurons and neural networks located in specific areas of the brain and utilizing specific neurotransmitters. There exists both a global (hypothalamic/brainstem) and local regulation of sleep. Global wake-promoting systems activate the thalamocortical circuits. Coordinated removal of arousal systems leads to hyperpolarization of thalamocortical neurons (wake-sleep switch). Activation of VLPO (GABA) neurons promotes sleep. Pontine cholinergic neurons generate REM sleep. With local sleep, neocortical areas that are most active during waking demonstrate greater local EEG slow wave activity during sleep. Regions of local sleep then phase-locks with other local sleep regions, eventually leading to synchronization of these semi-autonomous units and creating "global sleep."

	Description
Neural systems generating wakefulness	Include the ascending reticular formation in the medulla, pons and midbrain [neurotransmitter: glutamate], basal forebrain [PPT and LDT nuclei; acetylcholine], hypothalamus [hypocretin], locus coeruleus [norepinephrine], tuberomammillary nucleus [histamine], substantia nigra [dopamine] and raphe nuclei [serotonin]. There are two major pathways of the ascending reticular formation, namely the *dorsal* thalamocortical pathway (reticular formation → thalamus [midline and intralaminar thalamic nuclei] → cerebral cortex) and *ventral* pathway (reticular formation → posterior hypothalamus and subthalamus → basal forebrain → cerebral cortex). There are additional inputs to the ventral pathway, including basal forebrain (GABA and acetylcholine), dorsal raphe and median raphe nuclei (serotonin), lateral hypothalamus

	(hypocretin and melanin-concentrating hormone), locus coeruleus (norepinephrine), tuberomamillary nucleus (histamine) and ventral periaqueductal gray (dopamine).
Neural systems generating NREM sleep	Includes VLPO area of hypothalamus (GABA and galanin), medial preoptic nucleus (GABA and nitric oide), basal forebrain (GABA and adenosine) and thalamus. Activation of VLPO promotes both NREM and REM sleep. Projections to (a) ascending systems inhibit wake, (b) monoamine systems control NREM sleep, and (c) cholinergic pontine tegmentum control REM sleep. Medial preoptic nucleus project to hypocretin, serotonin and norepinephrine neurons. Sleep spindles originate in the reticular thalamic system [GABA] (interaction between thalamic relay neurons and reticular nucleus). Delta waves originate in the cortex and thalamus (interaction between thalamus and corticothalamic projections).
Neural systems generating REM sleep	REM sleep is associated with activation of "REM-on" neurons (cholinergic [caudal mesencephalon and rostral pons, including LDT and PPT nuclei]) and inhibition of "REM-off" neurons (noradrenergic [locus coeruleus], serotonergic [dorsal raphe] and histaminergic [tuberomammillary nuclei]). REM sleep develops with reduction/cessation of discharge of norepinephrine, serotonin and histamine, and loss of inhibition of LDT/PPT. LDT/PPT has (a) ascending projections that produce EEG desynchrony as well as (b) descending projections that are responsible for muscle atonia. Other neural systems that are involved with REM sleep are non-cholinergic and non-monoamine systems, GABA neurons, melanin-concentrating neurons and hypocretin neurons.

Wake-active systems interact with sleep-active systems in the VLPO (GABA) and PPT/LDT (acetylcholine). There exist bidirectional reciprocal inhibitory interactions between VLPO and monoaminergic (histamine, serotonin and norepinephrine) neurons (wake-sleep switch). Activation of VLPO produces coordinated inhibition of multiple arousal systems and, thus, promotes sleep.

Wake, REM sleep and NREM sleep involves the depolarization and hyperpolarization of thalamocortical circuits. Depolarization (due to activity of acetylcholine [PPT/LDT], norepinephrine, histamine, glutamate, hypocretin and/or serotonin neurons) causes *tonic firing* of the thalamic and neocortical neurons during wake or REM sleep producing a low voltage mixed frequency (desynchronized) EEG pattern. Hyperpolarization (due to removal/deactivation of excitatory inputs from wake-promoting systems, and loss of sensory transmission via the thalamus to the cortex) leads to inhibition of low voltage, mixed frequency EEG activity and to unmasking of oscillating synchronized EEG waveforms (sleep spindles and slow wave activity) between thalamic, cortical and thalamocortical neurons. Thus, the transition from wake/REM sleep to NREM sleep involves a switch from high frequency tonic firing (desynchronized EEG activity) to low frequency rhythmic burst discharge (synchronized EEG activity).

Sleep-wake regulation

Two basic intrinsic factors interact to regulate the timing and consolidation of sleep and wake, namely *sleep homeostasis (process S)*, which is dependent on the sleep-wake cycle; and *circadian rhythm (process C)*, which is idependent of the sleep-wake cycle. These two processes influence sleep latency, duration and quality. A third process, *sleep inertia (process W)* or period of relative confusion, disorientation and sleepiness shortly after awakening, can also influence waking behavior and performance. Sleep inertia is greatest following awakenings during the biological night. Lastly, timing of sleep is also determined by behavioral influences (e.g., social activities and work schedules).

	Description
Circadian rhythm	Naturally occurring circadian rhythms *free-run* at a genetically determined frequency, which is generally slightly over 24 hours (most commonly about 24.2 hours) in the absence of environmental time cues. *Entrainment* adjusts and synchronizes the endogenous circadian rhythms to the external 24-hour period, using environmental cues called *zeitgebers*. *Phase shifting* is the process whereby intrinsic circadian rhythms are shifted forward or backward in response to a zeitgeber.
Sleep homeostasis	An increase in sleep pressure that is related to the duration of prior wakefulness (i.e., the longer a person is awake, the sleepier one becomes). Sleep pressure declines following a sufficient duration of sleep.

Circadian neurosystem

Circadian rhythms are controlled by transcription-translation positive and negative feedback loops involving positive, negative and regulatory components (clock genes and their protein products). Positive components include *Clock* and *Bmal1*, negative components are *Period* and *Cryptochrome*, and *Casein kinase 1 epsilon* is a regulatory component. It is likely that other genes may be involved.

The SCN in the anterior hypothalamus (above the optic chiasm) is the master circadian rhythm generator in mammals. Its activity is independent of the environment, firing more frequently during the daytime than at night. Actions of the SCN include promotion of wakefulness during the day and consolidation of sleep during the night. There are several afferent inputs, both photic and non-photic, to the SCN, including (a) main photic pathway (retina ganglion cells containing the photopigment, melanopsin → retinohypothalamic tract → SCN) and (b) alternate photic pathway (thalamic intergeniculate leaflet of the lateral geniculate nuclei → geniculohypothalamic tract → SCN). The SCN, in turn, has efferent projections to the VLPO, lateral hypothalamus, paraventricular nucleus, pineal gland (medial forebrain bundle → spinal cord intermediolateral gray column neurons → superior cervical ganglion → pineal gland), and a number of organ systems.

Melatonin is a physiological marker of biological night, and is synthesized and released by the pineal gland. Secretion is greatest during the (biologic) night, least during the (biologic) day, and is inhibited by light exposure. Melatonin phase delays circadian sleep-wake rhythms when taken in the morning, and phase advances circadian sleep-wake rhythms when given in the afternoon or early evening. Melatonin also possesses mild hypnotic properties.

Physiologic changes during sleep

The sleep state is accompanied by significant changes in most organ systems. It is important to distinguish physiologic changes occurring during sleep from those that are secondary to circadian influences.

	NREM sleep
Central nervous system	Cerebral blood flow decreases during NREM sleep and increases during REM sleep.
Autonomic system	↓ Sympathetic activity and ↑ parasympathetic activity during NREM sleep and tonic REM sleep. Transient ↑ sympathetic activity during phasic REM sleep.
Respiratory system	*Control of respiration*: Both metabolic (i.e., pH, PaO_2 and $PaCO_2$) and behavioral control during wake but only metabolic control during sleep. *Hypoxic and hypercapnic ventilatory responses*: ↓ During NREM sleep (compared to wake) and ↓↓ during REM sleep. *Blood gas parameters*: Compared to wake, ↓ PaO_2 by 2-12 mmHg, ↓ SaO_2 by 2% and ↑ $PaCO_2$ by 2-8 mmHg during sleep. *UA dilator muscle tone*: ↓ During NREM sleep (compared to wake) and ↓↓ during REM sleep. *Activity of accessory muscles of respiration*: ↓ During NREM sleep (compared to wake) and ↓↓ during REM sleep. *Tidal volume and minute ventilation*: ↓ During sleep (compared to wake). *Respiratory patterns during sleep*: Periodic breathing with periods of hypopnea and hyperpnea during N1 sleep; stable and regular frequency and amplitude of respiration during N3 sleep; and irregular pattern of respiration (variable RR and TV) during REM sleep.
Cardiovascular system	*NREM sleep* (compared to wake): ↓ HR, ↓ CO, ↓ BP and =/↓ SVR. *Tonic REM sleep* (compared

	to NREM sleep): ↓ HR, ↓ CO, ↓ BP and ↓ SVR. *Phasic REM sleep* (compared to NREM and tonic REM sleep): ↑ HR, ↑ CO, ↑ BP and ↑ SVR. *During arousals and awakenings:* ↑ HR, ↑ CO, ↑ BP and ↑ SVR. Nighttime systolic BP is commonly about 10% less than daytime systolic BP ("dipping" phenomenon).
Gastrointestinal system	↓ Swallowing rate and salivary production; ↓ esophageal motility; ↓ gastric emptying; ↓ intestinal motility; ↑ rectal motor activity; and ↓ anal canal pressure.
Renal system	↑ Water reabsorption; ↓ GFR; and ↑ renin (during NREM sleep) and ADH.
Genito-urinary system	Penile tumescence (men) and clitoral tumescence and vaginal engorgement (women).
Endocrine system	*Growth hormone:* Release occurs primarily during N3 sleep. *Prolactin:* Secretion increases during N3 sleep and decreases during REM sleep. *TSH:* Secretion is linked to both sleep and circadian rhythms; secretion is low during the daytime, increases during the night, peaks prior to sleep onset, is inhibited by sleep, and increases with awakenings. *Cortisol:* Secretion is linked primarily to the circadian rhythm rather than to sleep; levels begin to rise about 2 hours prior to awakening (peak levels at 8-9 AM), decline thereafter (nadir at 12 AM), and are suppressed by sleep (especially N3). *Melatonin:* Levels rise in the evening, peak in the early morning (between 2-5 AM), and decline thereafter, even if no sleep occurs during the night; synthesis and secretion of melatonin are suppressed by light exposure. *Insulin:* ↓ Levels during sleep. *Leptin:* Greater secretion at night (highest levels from 12 PM to 4 AM and lowest levels from 1-2 PM). *Ghrelin:* ↑ Levels during the first part of the night and ↓ during the second part

	of the night and during the day; sleep may inhibit ghrelin release.
Musculoskeletal system	Skeletal muscle relaxation (hypotonia or atonia) and inhibition of deep tendon reflexes.
Pupillary changes	Pupillary constriction during tonic REM sleep and dilatation during phasic REM sleep.
Immunity	Pro-inflammatory cytokines (IL-1β and TNF-α) enhance NREM sleep and EEG slow wave activity, and reduce REM sleep. Anti-inflammatory cytokines (IL-4, IL-10 and transforming growth factor-beta) suppress sleep.
Thermoregulation	Core body temperature peaks in the late afternoon and early evening (6-8 PM) and falls at the onset of sleep. Temperature nadir occurs about 2-4 hours prior to usual wake time (4-5 AM). Changes in thermoregulation during sleep include ↓ core body temperature; ↓ thermal set point; ↓ thermoregulatory responses to thermal challenges; ↓ metabolic heat production [heat production from shivering is lost during REM sleep]; and ↑ heat loss [due to sweating and peripheral vasodilatation].
Metabolism	*NREM*: ↓ compared to wake. *REM*: ↑/= compared to NREM sleep.
Dreaming	Compared to REM sleep-related dreams that tend to be more complex and irrational, NREM dreams are generally simpler and relatively more realistic.

Sleep deprivation

Vulnerability to SD varies within individuals across time and between individuals. Furthermore, progressive SD correspondingly increases differences in performance across time in a person (*state instability*) as well as between different persons (*differential vulnerability*). Thus, there is intra- and inter-individual variability in tolerance to, and performance during, SD. The physiological and neurocognitive consequences of total SD appear to differ in some ways from those of chronic sleep restriction. The consequences of sleep deprivation are listed in the following table.

	Description
General	↑ Mortality (with habitual TST either < 6.5 or > 7.5 hours per night); ↑ sleepiness; ↓ vigilance and alertness; ↓ vigor; and ↑ fatigue.
Central nervous system	↓ Pain tolerance; ↓ seizure threshold; hyperactive gag and deep tendon reflexes; nystagmus, ptosis and sluggish corneal reflexes; slurring of speech; tremors; and ↓ motor skills.
Autonomic system	↑ Sympathetic activity.
Cognition	↓ Cognitive performance (↓ learning and ↑ memory lapses); ↓ attention and concentration; ↓ working memory and several components of executive function; ↓ information processing and decision-making; slowing of response/reaction time; and hyperactivity (in children).
Respiratory system	↓ FEV_1, FVC and ventilatory responsiveness.
Cardiovascular system	↑ BP and HR variability; and ↑ risk of coronary events (if TST is < 6 hours).

Endocrine system	↑ Cortisol, ACTH (evening levels), ghrelin and TSH (evening levels); ↓ GH, leptin activity and prolactin; and ↑ insulin resistance (↓ glucose tolerance) and risk of type 2 DM.
Metabolism	Increase in hunger, appetite (preference for salty, sweet and starchy foods) and caloric intake. Weight gain (weight loss in late stages of profound SD) and increased risk of obesity.
Immune system	↑ Proinflammatory markers (IL-1, IL-6, CRP and TNF-α); ↓ natural killer cell activity; ↓ antibody titers to influenza and hepatitis A vaccinations acutely; ↓ febrile response to endotoxin; and ↓ resistance to infection (presence of bacteria in sterile areas of the body).
Ocular changes	↓ Saccadic velocity; ↑ slow eye movements; and ↑ frequency of slow eyelid closures.
Behavioral and psychiatric effects	Negative impact on mood; and transient remission of major depressive disorder (in ≈ 50% of patients).
Societal impact	↑ Medical errors; ↑ motor vehicle accidents; and ↑ missed days of work.
PSG features	↓ SOL (also seen in the MSLT and MWT); ↑ TST; ↓ N2; ↑ slow wave EEG activity; ↓ sleep spindles; and ↓ REM SL. During recovery sleep, ↑ N3 (1st night after SD) and ↑ R (2nd night after SD).
Waking EEG features	Shift to slower EEG frequencies (theta [4-7 Hz] and delta [< 4 Hz] waves).

Polysomnography

PSG involves the continuous and simultaneous recording of several physiologic variables during sleep. PSG is indicated for the diagnosis of SRBD; PAP titration for SRBD; pre-operative assessment prior to UA surgery for OSA or snoring; follow-up after UA surgery, dental devices or significant weight loss (in obese persons) for OSA; diagnosis of narcolepsy (followed by MSLT on the day following PSG); diagnosis of PLMD; evaluation of unexplained EDS; evaluation of atypical or injurious parasomnias (with additional EEG derivations and video recording); and evaluation of suspected nocturnal seizures (with additional EEG leads and video recording).

Portable sleep apnea testing (PSAT), as an alternative to PSG, is indicated (a) for persons with a high pre-test probability of OSA; (b) as follow-up assessment to determine response to therapy for OSA; or (c) in instances when PSG is unavailable or unsafe. It is not recommended for (a) persons with significant medical comorbidities, such as CHF or moderate-to-severe pulmonary disease; (b) persons with suspected CSA or narcolepsy; or (c) as screening of asymptomatic persons.

The polygraph equipment

A polygraph, consisting of a series of AC and DC amplifiers and filters, records several physiologic variables during sleep. Amplification refers to the augmentation of biopotential differences from 2 sources to permit better visualization. A derivation is the difference in voltage between 2 electrodes. It can be either *bipolar* (two standard electrodes are matched to each other) or *referential* (a standard electrode is matched to a reference electrode). High-frequency (fast) physiologic variables (e.g., EEG, EOG, EMG and ECG) are recorded using *AC amplifiers*. Low-frequency (slow) physiologic variables (e.g., SaO_2 and CPAP levels) are recorded using *DC amplifiers*. Airflow and respiratory effort are recorded using either AC or DC amplifiers. A third type of filter, the notch filter, is used to attenuate 60 Hz electrical interferences from other AC devices.

Fall time constant is the duration required for a square wave voltage to decay to 63% of its original maximum amplitude. Fall time constant is inversely related to the low frequency filter setting. Polarity refers to the direction of deflection of waveforms (i.e., a positive voltage/polarity causes a downward deflection, whereas a negative voltage/polarity causes an upward deflection). Sampling rate is the frequency at which a signal is converted from an analog to digital format. An acceptable sampling rate is commonly 2-6 X the frequency of a signal. Lower than optimal sampling rates can cause signal distortion (i.e., aliasing).

Basic steps in performing a polysomnogram

(a) A sleep diary is completed for 2 weeks before the study. PSG is performed during the patient's customary bedtime. (b) Questionnaires (including measures of sleepiness) are completed prior to the start of the study. (c) Placement of electrodes and sensors. Each channel is provided appropriate settings for sensitivity, and high- and low-frequency filters. (d) Biocalibrations are performed. Patients are asked to perform certain actions (e.g., look up and down, or breathe in and out) to check the integrity of the electrodes and amplifiers. (e) Study is started. Time when recording started ("lights out") is noted. (f) Monitoring and observation. Correction of artifacts, if present. Titration of PAP, if indicated. (g) Study is ended. The time the study ended ("lights on") is recorded. (h) Biocalibrations are repeated. (i) Post-study questionnaires are completed.

Variables recorded during polysomnography

Variables recorded during sleep include EEG, EOG, EMG, ECG, airflow, snoring, thoracic and abdominal movement, and SaO_2. Other sensors that may be used during PSG include esophageal pressure monitors, $PetCO_2$, $PtcCO_2$, PAP level, additional EEG channels (for evaluation of suspected nocturnal seizures), video monitoring (for evaluation of suspected parasomnias or seizures), and esophageal pH sensors (for evaluation of suspected GER).

	Description
Electroencephalography	Placement of EEG electrodes is based on the International 10-20 system. Each electrode is provided with a letter that represents the corresponding region of the brain (e.g., frontal [F], central [C], occipital [O] and mastoid [M]) and a numerical subscript (odd numbers for left-sided electrodes, even numbers for right-sided electrodes, and "Z" for midline electrodes). Recommended electrode placements are F4M1, C4M1 and O2M1. The voltage recorded from EEG electrodes originates from the summed potential activity of cortical neurons. Frequencies of EEG waves [Hz] are delta (< 4), theta (4-7), alpha (8-13) and beta (> 13). *Delta waves* have high amplitudes (peak to peak of > 75 μV). Amplitude of *alpha waves* is generally < 50 μV in adults. *K complex* is a high-amplitude, biphasic wave (an initial sharp negative deflection immediately followed by a positive high-voltage slow wave) with duration of ≥ 0.5 seconds and with a frequency of < 2 Hz. *Saw-tooth waves* are theta waves with notched waveforms and that occur during REM sleep. *Sleep spindles* are brief oscillations with frequencies of 12-14 Hz lasting 0.5-1.5 seconds and amplitudes that are generally < 50 μV.

Vertex sharp deflections are sharp negative waves with amplitudes < 250 µV.

Electro-oculography	Records the difference in potentials (dipole) between the cornea (positively charged) and the retina (negatively charged). This dipole changes with eye movements. A positive voltage (downward deflection) is recorded when the eye moves toward an electrode, and a negative voltage (upward deflection) accompanies an eye movement away from an electrode. Recommended electrode placements are E1M2 and E2M2 (where E1 = 1 cm below the left outer canthus, E2 = 1 cm above the right outer canthus, and M2 = right mastoid process). Conjugate eye movements create *out-of-phase* deflections in the two EOG channels. EEG artifacts produce *in-phase* deflections. There are two general patterns of eye movements, namely *slow rolling eye movements* that occur during relaxed drowsiness with closed eyes, N1 sleep or brief awakenings, and disappear during N2 sleep; and *rapid eye movements* that occur during waking with open eyes (eye blinks) or during REM sleep.
Electromyography (chin)	Three electrodes are used and are located (a) midline, 1 cm above the inferior edge of the mandible; and (b, c) 2 cm to the right or left of midline and 2 cm below the inferior edge of the mandible. Derivation consists of either one of the electrodes below the mandible referred to the electrode placed above the mandible.
Electrocardiography	A single modified lead II with electrodes placed below the right clavicle near the sternum and over the lateral chest wall at the left 6th or 7th intercostal space.
Measuring airflow	Pneumotachography is the reference standard for detecting obstructive apnea-hypopneas.

	The recommended techniques for identifying apneas and hypopneas are the *oronasal thermal sensor* and *nasal air pressure transducer*, respectively. With nasal pressure monitoring, obstructive respiratory events are associated with a plateau (flattening) of the inspiratory flow signal whereas central respiratory events are associated with reduced but rounded signals.
Measuring respiratory effort	Recommended sensors for measuring respiratory effort are *esophageal manometry* or *inductance plethysmography*. Measurement of respiratory effort is important to distinguish obstructive, central and mixed apneas.
Measuring oxygenation and ventilation	Recommended sensor for O_2 saturation is pulse *oximetry*. Recommended sensors for alveolar hypoventilation are *$PtcCO_2$* or *$PetCO_2$*.
Identifying snoring	Snoring can be detected using a microphone.
Electromyography (anterior tibialis)	Electrodes placed over the anterior tibialis of both legs are used to detect PLMS. Additional electrodes can be placed over the upper extremities (extensor digitorum communis) to identify RBD.

Technical specifications for PSG electrodes and sensors

Strict adherence to recommended parameters for sampling rates, high and low frequency filters, and impedance for electrodes and sensors during PSG is essential in order to acquire optimal recordings for sleep stage and event scoring and study interpretation.

	EEG and EOG	*EMG and snoring*	*ECG*	*Respiration*	*Oximetry*
Desirable sampling rate (Hz)	500	500	500		25
Minimal sampling rate (Hz)	200	200	200		10
High frequency filter (Hz)	35	100	70	15	
Low frequency filter (Hz)	0.3	10	0.3	0.1	
Maximum impedance (K ohms)	5				

For airflow, nasal pressure, esophageal pressure and chest/abdominal movements, desirable and minimal sampling rates are 100 and 25 Hz, respectively.

Scoring sleep in adults and children

PSG data are divided into 30-second time periods or epochs. The standard sleep study paper speed is 10 mm/second (30 cm per epoch page). Each epoch is assigned a single sleep stage that comprises the greatest percentage of the epoch. Rules for scoring sleep in children apply to infants $\geq$ 2 months post-term.

Normal sleep in an adult is characterized by short sleep latency (< 15 minutes), high sleep efficiency (> 95%), and few and relatively brief awakenings. Sleep is typically entered into through NREM sleep. The period from NREM stages 1-3 to REM sleep is called a *sleep cycle*. There are commonly 3-5 NREM-REM sleep cycles during the night, each occurring every 90-120 minutes in adults. N3 sleep predominates in the 1st half of the night whereas REM sleep percentage is greater during the 2nd half of the night.

	Adults	*Children*
Stage Wake *(see page 185)*	> 50% of the epoch has alpha EEG waves over the occipital region with eye closure. If alpha waves are absent, any of the following is present, namely conjugate vertical eye blinks (0.5-2 Hz), reading eye movements (conjugate slow movement followed by a rapid movement in the opposite direction), or voluntary rapid open eye movements. Usually relatively high chin EMG tone.	> 50% of the epoch contains alpha or dominant posterior EEG rhythm.

Stage N1 (see page 186)	Alpha EEG waves are replaced by low amplitude, mixed frequency (4-7 Hz) waves that occupy > 50% of the epoch. In persons who do not generate alpha waves, the start of one of the following: theta (4-7 Hz) waves with slowing of background EEG activity by ≥ 1 Hz compared to stage W; vertex sharp waves with duration of < 0.5 seconds; or presence of slow eye movements. No rapid eye movements, K complexes and sleep spindles are present. Tonic chin EMG levels are typically lower than during relaxed wakefulness.	Alpha or dominant posterior EEG rhythm is replaced by low amplitude, mixed frequency (4-7 Hz) waves occupying > 50% of the epoch. In those who do not generate a dominant posterior rhythm, the start of one of the following: 4-7 Hz waves with slowing of the background activity by ≥ 1-2 Hz compared to stage W; vertex sharp waves; slow eye movements; rhythmic anterior theta activity; hypnagogic hypersynchrony; or diffuse or occipital-predominant high amplitude 3-5 Hz rhythmic activity.
Stage N2 (see page 187)	The start of stage N2 is defined by the presence of K complexes (not associated with arousals) or sleep spindles during the 1st half of the epoch or during the last half of the previous epoch if criteria for stage N3 are absent. The continuation of stage N2 is defined by the presence of low amplitude, mixed frequency EEG rhythms, and if the epoch contains, or is preceded, by K complexes (not associated with arousals) or sleep	Same as adult scoring rules.

	spindles. Scoring of stage N2 is terminated when the epoch is scored as W, N3 or R; or when arousals or major body movements are followed by N1 (low amplitude, mixed frequency EEG).	
Stage N3 *(see page 188)*	≥ 20% of the epoch (≥ 6 seconds) is occupied by slow wave (0.5-2 Hz and > 75 μV) EEG activity over the frontal regions.	Same as adult scoring rules.
Stage REM *(see page 189)*	Presence of all of the following: low amplitude, mixed frequency activity in the EEG; rapid eye movements in the EOG; and low tone (lowest level in the study or at least no higher than the other sleep stages) in the chin EMG. The continuation of stage R is defined by the presence of (a) low amplitude, mixed frequency EEG activity, (b) low chin EMG tone, (c) no K complexes or sleep spindles in epochs that either contain rapid eye movements or that are preceded by stage R, and (d) no arousals or major body movements followed by slow eye movements.	Same as adult scoring rules.

Stage NREM		If K complexes, sleep spindles and slow wave activity are absent in all epochs of NREM sleep.

Major body movements are defined by the presence of movements or muscle artifact that obscures the EEG for > 50% of the epoch. An epoch with a major body movement is scored the same stage as the epoch that follows it, but is scored as stage W if (a) alpha rhythm is present or (b) if it is preceded, or followed, by a stage W epoch.

Scoring sleep in newborn infants

Sleep scoring in newborns also follows an "epoch" approach using behavior, respiration, EEG, EOG and EMG data. Sleep is classified as either active REM sleep or quiet sleep. The term "intermediate sleep" is used when epochs do not fully meet criteria for active or quiet sleep.

	Stage wake	Stage active (REM) sleep	Stage quiet sleep
Behavior	Eyes open, visible movements and vocalizations	Eyes closed, visible movements (facial grimaces, smiles or movements of body and limbs) and vocalizations	Eyes closed and no body movements
Respiration	Variable	Irregular	Regular
EEG	Mixed slow wave (theta) pattern with occasional beta and delta waveforms	Low-voltage irregular pattern or mixed pattern	High-voltage slow pattern, trace alternant pattern or mixed pattern
EOG	Waking eye movements	Positive	Negative
EMG	Sustained tone with bursts of phasic activity	Low	High

Respiration is classified *regular* (rate varies < 20 breaths per minute) or *irregular* (rate varies > 20 breaths per minute). EEG is classified as *high-voltage slow pattern* (continuous, medium- to high-amplitude [50-150 μV] waveforms; frequencies from 0.5-4 Hz), *low-voltage irregular pattern* (low-amplitude [14-35 μV] waveforms; frequencies from 5-8 Hz), *trace alternant pattern* (bursts of slow [0.5-3 Hz] high-amplitude waves, fast low-amplitude waves, and sharp waves [2-4 Hz] lasting several seconds interspersed with periods of relative quiescence [mixed frequency waveforms] lasting 4-8 seconds, or *mixed pattern* (high- and low-voltage waveforms). EOG is classified as either *positive* (rapid eye movements are present) or *negative* (no rapid eye movements). *EMG* is classified as either *high* (tonic activity occupies > half of epoch) or *low* (tonic activity occupies < half of epoch).

Scoring arousals

NREM arousals require changes in EEG only. REM arousals require changes in EEG and EMG.

	Required changes
EEG	Abrupt EEG frequency shift (to alpha, theta or > 16 Hz, but not spindles) ≥ 3 seconds and preceded by ≥ 10 seconds of stable sleep.
EMG	Increase in chin EMG tone ≥ 1 second.

Scoring respiratory events

Accurate scoring of respiratory events is essential as is determining if these phenomena are pathologic or normal sleep-related physiologic events. Pediatric rules apply to children < 18 yrs of age.

	Adult	Pediatric
Apnea (see page 190 and 191)	Decrease in peak thermal sensor amplitude by ≥ 90% of baseline for a duration of ≥ 10 seconds. (Note: ≥ 9 seconds in a row must meet the 90% amplitude change criterion). Events can either be obstructive (inspiratory effort is present throughout the entire event); central (inspiratory effort is absent throughout the entire event); or mixed (absent inspiratory effort in the initial part of the event followed by inspiratory effort). Complex sleep apnea refers to the development or worsening of central apneas during CPAP titration or treatment for OSA.	≥ 90% fall in signal amplitude lasting ≥ 2 missed breaths. Events can either be obstructive, central or mixed.
Hypopnea (see page 191)	Decrease in nasal pressure amplitude by ≥ 30% of baseline for a duration of ≥ 10 seconds accompanied by ≥ 4% O_2 desaturation. (Note: ≥ 9	≥ 50% reduction in nasal pressure amplitude compared to baseline, associated with an arousal,

	seconds in a row must meet the 30% amplitude change criterion).	awakening, or $\geq$ 3% O_2 desaturation, lasting for a duration of $\geq$ 2 missed breaths.
Respiratory effort-related arousal	Breaths associated with increasing respiratory effort or flattening of the nasal pressure waveform, with a duration of $\geq$ 10 seconds, followed by an arousal. Does not meet criteria for either apnea or hypopnea.	When using a nasal pressure sensor, there is a reduction in sensor signal to < 50% of baseline levels, associated with flattening of the waveform, snoring, increase in $PtcCO_2$ or $PetCO_2$, or visible increase in work of breathing lasting $\geq$ 2 breath cycles.
Hypoventilation	$\geq$ 10 mmHg increase in $PaCO_2$ during sleep compared to supine wake values.	$PtcCO_2$ or $PetCO_2$ > 50 mmHg in > 25% of TST.
Cheyne Stokes respiration	$\geq$ 3 consecutive cycles of crescendo-decrescendo amplitude in respiration interrupted by apneic episodes *plus* either (a) duration of CSR of $\geq$ 10 consecutive minutes, or (b) $\geq$ 5 central apneas/hypopneas per hour of sleep.	
Periodic breathing		> 3 episodes of central apneas with duration of > 3 sec separated by $\leq$ 20 seconds of normal respiration.

Scoring movement events

Movements are not uncommon during sleep. Determining clinical significance requires a thorough and thoughtful assessment of both presenting history and PSG data.

	Description
Alternating leg muscle activation	≥ 4 EMG bursts, 0.5-3 Hz in frequency, alternating between legs with duration of 100-500 msec.
Bruxism *(see page 192)*	Increase in chin EMG activity that is ≥ 2 times above the background EMG tone, separated by ≥ 3 seconds of stable EMG. Episodes are either brief (0.25-2 seconds in duration occurring in a sequence of ≥ 3 episodes) or sustained (> 2 seconds in duration). There are ≥ 2 audible bruxism episodes per night.
Excessive fragmentary myoclonus	≥ 5 EMG bursts (each with a usual maximum duration of 150 msec) per minute occurring for ≥ 20 min of NREM sleep.
Hypnagogic foot tremor	≥ 4 EMG bursts, 0.3-4 Hz in frequency, with duration of 250-1000 msec.
Periodic limb movements of sleep	≥ 4 consecutive leg movements, each 0.5-10 seconds in duration with amplitude ≥ 8 μV above resting EMG tone. Period lengths (time from the start of one leg movement to the start of the next) are 5-90 seconds between consecutive movements. Leg movements are not scored if they are within 0.5 seconds before and after an apnea/hypopnea. Leg movements on different legs are counted as 1 movement if they are separated by < 5 seconds between movement onsets.

	Legs movements and arousals are considered to be related if they occur within 0.5 seconds of each other.
REM sleep behavior disorder	Sustained chin EMG muscle activity; excessive transient chin or limb EMG muscle activity; or both occurring during REM sleep.
Rhythmic movement disorder	≥ 4 individual movements, each with a frequency of 0.5-2 Hz and an amplitude ≥ 2 times above resting EMG tone.

Important cardiac arrhythmias

Proper ECG electrode application will reduce artifacts and facilitate cardiac rhythm recognition.

	Definition
Asystole	Cardiac pause > 3 seconds in duration (for patients ≥ 6 years old).
Sinus bradycardia	HR < 40 beats per minute (for patients ≥ 6 years old).
Sinus tachycardia	HR > 90 beats per minute (for adult patients). Sinus rates are faster in young children.
Narrow-complex tachycardia	HR > 100 beats per minute. At least 3 consecutive beats with QRS duration < 120 msec.
Wide-complex tachycardia	HR > 100 beats per minute. At least 3 consecutive beats with QRS duration ≥ 120 msec.
Atrial fibrillation	Irregularly irregular rhythm with no P waves.

PSG artifacts

Artifacts are unwanted recordings during PSG that arise either from faulty electrode placement, defective monitoring devices or amplifiers, or contamination by physiologic or environmental variables. Artifacts can be generalized (affecting several or most channels) or localized (limited to a single channel). *Generalized* artifacts suggest a defective reference electrode that is common to the affected channels. *Localized* artifacts suggest a defect in the specific electrode itself.

	Description	Cause/s	Corrective measure/s
60 Hz interference *(see page 192)*	Dense, square-shaped EEG tracing.	Due to (a) interference by 60 Hz electrical activity from power lines, (b) high and unequal electrode impedance, or (c) lead failure.	Fix electrode placement or change leads. Use 60 Hz filter as a last resort.
ECG artifact	Presence of ECG waveforms in non-ECG leads.	Contamination from ECG leads.	Fix electrode placement or change lead.
Electrode popping *(see page 193)*	Sudden, sharp, high-amplitude deflection.	Due to (a) pulling of electrode leads away from the skin by body movements or respiration, (b) patient	Fix electrode placement or change lead. Apply more electrode gel.

		lying on the electrode, (c) faulty electrode placement, or (d) drying out of the electrode gel.	
Sweat artifact *(see page 193)*	Slow undulating movements that are synchronous with respiration.	Due to alterations in electrode potentials by salt in sweat.	Decrease room temperature.

Definitions of polysomnographic parameters

Standard definitions of PSG terms are listed.

	Definition
Apnea index (AI)	Number of apneas per hour of sleep
Apnea-hypopnea index (AHI)	Number of apneas *plus* hypopneas per hour of sleep
Alpha-delta	Alpha waves occurring during N3 sleep
Arousal index	Number of arousals per hour of sleep
Bedtime	Time when a person gets into bed and attempts to fall asleep
Final awakening	Time when a person awakens for the final time
Lights out (LO)	Time when sleep recording starts
Lights on (LOn)	Time when sleep recording ends
Oxygen desaturation index (ODI)	Number of O_2 desaturation events per hour of sleep
Periodic limb movement index	Number of periodic limb movements per hour of sleep
REM sleep latency (REM SL)	Time in minutes from the onset of sleep to the first epoch of REM sleep.
Sleep efficiency (SE)	Ratio of TST to TIB [(TST X 100)/TIB]
Sleep onset latency (SOL)	Time from lights out to sleep onset (i.e., first epoch of any stage of sleep) [< 15-30 minutes in healthy adults]

Sleep onset REM period (SOREMP)	Occurrence of REM sleep within 10-15 minutes of sleep onset
Time in bed (TIB)	Duration of monitoring between "lights out" to "lights on"
Total sleep time (TST)	Sum of all sleep stages (NREM stages 1-3 sleep *plus* REM sleep) in minutes
Wake after sleep onset (WASO)	Time spent awake from sleep onset to final awakening

Other tests of sleep

Aside from PSG and PSAT, there are several other important tests relevant to clinical sleep medicine, including subjective and objective measures of sleepiness and alertness as well as techniques to identify patterns of sleep and waking.

	Description
Epworth sleepiness scale	Eight-item questionnaire that measures a person's general propensity to fall asleep in various situations in recent times, including (a) sitting and reading; (b) watching television; (c) sitting and inactive in a public place; (d) as a passenger in a car for an hour without a break; (e) lying down to rest in the afternoon; (f) sitting and talking to someone; (g) sitting quietly after lunch without drinking alcohol; and (h) stopped in a car for a few minutes in traffic. A person's chances of dozing are rated as 0 (never), 1 (slight chance), 2 (moderate chance) or 3 (high chance). An aggregate score of 0-9 is considered normal, whereas scores of ≥ 10 suggests that sleepiness is present and that sleep specialist advice is recommended.
Stanford sleepiness scale	Seven-point subjective measure of perception of sleepiness at a given time, ranging from "wide awake, vital and alert" to "unable to remain awake with sleep onset imminent".
Multiple sleep latency test	An objective measure of the physiologic tendency to fall asleep in quiet situations. Indicated for evaluation of unexplained EDS or suspected narcolepsy, and for distinguishing between narcolepsy and idiopathic hypersomnia.
	Adequate sleep duration and regular sleep-wake schedules should be maintained for ≥ 1-2

weeks prior to MSLT. Medications that can affect SOL and REM sleep (e.g., stimulants, hypnotics, sedatives, REM suppressants and opioids) should be discontinued for $\geq$ 2 weeks (or $\geq$ 5 times the half-life of the drug and its longest-acting metabolite) before the study. A nocturnal PSG should be performed immediately before an MSLT to exclude other causes of EDS (e.g., OSA or PLMD). An MSLT should not be performed after a split-night PSG. There should be an adequate duration of nocturnal sleep ($\geq$ 6 hours) during the preceding PSG. OSA, if present, should be adequately treated before performing an MSLT. If the patient uses PAP for OSA, it should be used during PSG and MSLT.

The study consists of 4-5 nap opportunities. Each nap trial is 20 minutes in duration, performed every 2 hours starting about 1.5-3 hours after awakening from the previous night's sleep. Smoking and stimulating activities should be stopped before each nap trial. Caffeine and vigorous physical activity should be avoided during the day of the study. A urine drug screen should be performed during test day. Standard leads include EEG, EOG, chin EMG and ECG. Standard biocalibrations are performed before and after each trial.

During the trial, the patient is asked to lie down in a comfortable position in a dark, quiet room, close his/her eyes and *try to fall asleep*. A nap trial is terminated after 20 minutes if no sleep is recorded. If sleep is recorded, the test is continued for an additional 15 minutes to allow REM sleep to occur. The test is stopped after the 1st epoch of unequivocal REM sleep; alternatively, the test may be continued for the entire additional 15 minutes. The patient is asked to get out of bed and to remain awake between nap trials. A shorter 4-nap test may be considered if ≥ 2 SOREMPs have already occurred during earlier nap trials, and if the mean SOL is abnormal (< 4 minutes for the initial 4 nap trials).

SOL is defined as the time from lights out to the onset of sleep (i.e., 1st epoch of any stage of sleep for clinical MSLT). If no sleep occurs during a nap trial, its SOL is recorded as 20 minutes. In addition, the occurrence of SOREMPs (> 15 seconds of REM sleep in a 30-second epoch) is determined for each nap trial. REM SL is the time from the 1st epoch of sleep to the beginning of the 1st epoch of REM sleep.

Short mean SOL suggests the presence of EDS. Mean sleep latencies (mean ± SD [minutes]) are as follows: (a) normal controls, 4-nap MSLT: 10 ± 4; (b) normal controls, 5-nap MSLT: 11 ± 5; (c) narcolepsy: 3 ± 3; and (d) idiopathic hypersomnia: 6 ± 3. Normative MLST parameters are not well established for children < 8 years of age.

Maintenance of wakefulness test	An objective measure of a person's ability to remain awake in quiet situations for a specified period of time. Indicated to assess an individual's ability to maintain wakefulness, and to assess response to treatment for EDS.

Consists of 4 nap opportunities performed at 2-hour intervals. A *40-minute* protocol for each nap is recommended. The 1st nap trial is started about 1.5-3 hrs after the person's customary wake time. The need for a PSG prior to MWT should be individualized as determined by the clinician.

During each nap trial, a person is asked to sit in bed in a semi-reclined position and in a dark, quiet room. The person is instructed to *try to stay awake* during the test. However, measures to stay awake (e.g., singing) are not allowed during nap trials. Use of tobacco, caffeine and stimulant agents should be avoided during test day. Drug screening may be considered. Standard leads include EEG, EOG and chin EMG. Standard biocalibrations are performed before and after each nap trial.

The nap trial is terminated if (a) unequivocal sleep occurs (i.e., 3 consecutive epochs of N1 sleep or 1 epoch of any other sleep stage); or (b) no sleep is recorded after 40 minutes. SOL is defined as the time from lights out to the first epoch of sleep (sleep onset) for each nap. SOL correlates with the ability to stay awake. A mean SOL < 8 minutes is considered abnormal; > 8 minutes but < 40 minutes is of uncertain significance; and = 40 minutes is considered normal and may provide an appropriate expectation for individuals who require the highest level of alertness for safety.

Actigraphy	A technique to determine periods of inactivity (rest or sleep) or activity using sensors that can detect movement. Movements are detected using accelerometers that are typically worn on the wrist. Data can be recorded over a period of several days. Movement data are summated for a specified epoch time, and each epoch is scored as either "active" or inactive" based on predetermined thresholds for activity counts. Data that can be obtained with actigraphy include total wake time, TST, SOL (if used with an event monitor to mark the time when a person desires to fall asleep), frequency of awakenings and WASO.

Indicated (a) to evaluate circadian rhythm sleep disorders [except for jet lag] and their response to therapy. It may also be considered (b) to aid in the diagnosis of insomnia, particularly paradoxical insomnia; (c) to evaluate response to therapy for insomnia; (d) to estimate sleep in persons with OSA when PSG or PSAT are not available; and (e) to define sleep and circadian patterns in persons with hypersomnia.

Actigraphy monitoring for evaluation of CRSDs should include ≥ 3 consecutive 24-hour periods over ≥ 7 days.

General patterns of sleep architecture

There are 3 general patterns of sleep architecture, namely (a) high sleep input pattern, (b) low sleep input pattern, and (c) circadian rhythm disorder patterns.

	PSG features	Cause/s	Specific syndromes
High sleep input pattern	↓ SOL, ↑ SE, ↑ TST and ↓ WASO	SD; disorders presenting with EDS; and use of sedating medications.	(a) Idiopathic hypersomnia; (b) insufficient sleep syndrome; (c) narcolepsy; and (d) recurrent hypersomnia.
Low sleep input pattern	↑ SOL, ↓ SE, ↓ TST and ↑ WASO	Disorders presenting with insomnia; and use of stimulant medications.	(a) Adjustment insomnia; (b) idiopathic insomnia; (c) inadequate sleep hygiene; (d) limit-setting sleep disorder; (e) medical, neurological or psychiatric disorders; (f) PLMD; (g) environmental sleep disorder; (h) psychophysiologic insomnia; (i) RLS; and (j) sleep onset association insomnia.
Circadian rhythm sleep patterns	Variable sleep architecture depending on whether PSG is performed		*Delayed sleep phase syndrome* – ↑ SOL and ↓ TST if PSG is performed during *conventional* sleep schedule; but normal sleep architecture if PSG is performed during *habitual* later sleep schedule. *Advanced sleep phase syndrome* – ↓ or normal

during the conventional or habitual sleep schedule.

SOL, ↓ TST, and early wake time if PSG is performed during *conventional* sleep schedule; but normal sleep architecture if PSG is performed during *habitual* earlier sleep schedule.

Irregular sleep-wake rhythm – Variable and disorganized pattern of sleep and wake if 24-hour PSG is performed over several days.

Free-running disorder – Progressively ↑ SOL and ↓ TST if PSG is recorded at a fixed time period daily over several days.

Jet lag – ↓ SE and ↑ WASO; ↑ SOL after eastward travel, and ↓ SOL after westward travel if a person follows habitual bedtime at destination.

Shift work disorder – ↓ SE and ↑ WASO.

Differential diagnoses of sleep complaints

Every sleep-related symptom has a diverse differential diagnosis. Furthermore, many patients present with more than a single sleep complaint, thus, further complicating diagnosis.

Complaint	Syndrome/s
Chronic hypersomnia	(a) CRSDs; (b) idiopathic hypersomnia; (c) insufficient sleep syndrome; (d) long sleeper [after conventional sleep duration]; (e) medical, neurological and psychiatric disorders; (f) medication or substance use or withdrawal; (g) narcolepsy; (h) OSA and CSA; (i) PLMD; (j) post-traumatic hypersomnia [head injury]; and (k) recurrent hypersomnia.
Recurrent hypersomnia	(a) Bipolar disorder; (b) complex partial seizures; (c) DSPS [severe]; (d) FRD; (e) frequent jet travel; (f) idiopathic recurring stupor; (g) ISWR; (h) Kleine-Levin syndrome; (i) medication or substance use; (j) menstrual-associated hypersomnia; (k) metabolic encephalopathy; (l) poor sleep hygiene; (m) poor and irregular PAP therapy compliance for OSA; (n) seasonal affective disorder; and (o) SWD.
Transient insomnia	(a) Acute stressors; (b) jet lag; (c) medication use/withdrawal; and (d) SWD.
Chronic insomnia	(a) Altitude insomnia; (b) CRSDs; (c) environmental sleep disorder; (d) food allergy insomnia; (e) idiopathic insomnia; (f) inadequate sleep hygiene; (g) limit-setting sleep disorder; (h) medical, neurological and psychiatric disorders; (i) medication or substance use/withdrawal; (j) menstruation, pregnancy and menopause; (k)

	nightmares; (l) nocturnal leg cramps; (m) paradoxical insomnia; (n) PLMD; (o) psychophysiologic insomnia; (p) RLS; (q) sleep apnea [central or obstructive]; (r) sleep-onset association disorder; and (s) toxin-induced sleep disorder.
Sleep-onset insomnia (in children)	(a) Adjustment sleep disorder; (b) anxiety disorders; (c) ADHD; (d) bedtime resistance; (e) colic; (f) DSPS; (g) environmental sleep disorder; (h) food allergy insomnia; (i) inadequate sleep hygiene; (j) limit-setting sleep disorder; (k) medical disorders; (l) mood disorders; (m) nighttime fears [fear of darkness or being left alone]; (n) PTSD; (o) psychophysiologic insomnia; (p) RLS; (q) separation anxiety; (r) sleep-onset association disorder; and (s) variable sleep schedules.
Sleep-maintenance insomnia (in children)	(a) Colic; (b) inadequate sleep hygiene; (c) medical disorders; (d) OSA; (e) parasomnias [nightmares]; (f) PLMD; and (g) psychophysiologic insomnia.
Sleep-onset insomnia (general)	(a) Adjustment sleep disorder; (b) altitude insomnia; (c) CRSDs; (d) environmental sleep disorder; (e) idiopathic insomnia; (f) inadequate sleep hygiene; (g) medication use [stimulants] or withdrawal [hypnotic agents]; (h) paradoxical insomnia; (i) psychiatric disorders; (j) psychophysiologic insomnia; and (k) RLS.
Sleep-maintenance insomnia (general)	(a) Alcohol [withdrawal from]; (b) idiopathic insomnia; (c) medical, neurological and psychiatric disorders; (d) medication use (stimulants) or withdrawal [hypnotic agents]; (e) parasomnias; (f) PLMD; (g) psychophysiologic insomnia; and (h) sleep apnea [central or obstructive].

Terminal insomnia (early morning awakening)	(a) Alcohol [withdrawal from]; (b) ASPS; (c) depression; (d) jet lag [following westward travel]; and (e) withdrawal from short-acting hypnotic agents.
Persistently short nocturnal sleep duration	(a) Fatal familial insomnia; (b) idiopathic insomnia; (c) inadequate sleep hygiene; (d) manic phase of bipolar disorder; (e) polyphasic sleep with frequent daytime napping; (f) psychophysiologic insomnia; (g) short sleeper; and (h) stimulant use or abuse.
Sleeping better when away from home	(a) Psychophysiologic insomnia; (b) environmental sleep disorder; and (c) reverse "first-night" effect.
Vivid and disturbed dreaming	(a) Alcohol (withdrawal from); (b) isolated sleep paralysis; (c) medication and substance use (e.g., beta-blockers); (d) nightmare; (e) nocturnal panic attack; (f) OSA; (g) PTSD; (h) RBD; (i) schizophrenia; and (j) terrifying hypnagogic hallucination.
Unusual behavior or activity during sleep	(a) Confusional arousal; (b) malingering; (c) medication, substance or alcohol use; (d) nightmare; (e) nocturnal paroxysmal dystonia; (f) nocturnal psychogenic dissociative discorder; (g) nocturnal seizure; (h) OSA; (i) panic attack; (j) PLMD; (k) PTSD; (l) RBD; (m) rhythmic movement disorder; (n) sleep terror; and (o) sleepwalking.
Nighttime automatic behavior	(a) Dissociative and fugue-like states; (b) malingering; (c) medication, substance or alcohol use; (d) narcolepsy; (e) OSA; (f) parasomnias; (g) seizure (especially partial complex); and (h) SD.
Sleep paralysis	(a) Catatonia; (b) familial (X-linked dominant) paralysis; (c) isolated sleep paralysis; (d) narcolepsy; (e) seizure (atonic); (f) SD; and (g) transient (hyperkalemic or hypokalemic)

paralysis.

Nocturnal limb movements	(a) Fragmentary myoclonus; (b) neurodegenerative disorders (e.g., PD); (c) nocturnal seizure; (d) OSA-related arousal; (e) PLMS; (f) phasic movements during REM sleep; (g) RBD; (h) rhythmic movement disorder; and (i) sleep start.
Body movements at sleep onset	(a) PLMS; (b) propriospinal myoclonus; (c) RLS; (d) rhythmic movement disorder; and (e) sleep start.
Sound production	(a) Bruxism; (b) catathrenia; (c) confusional arousal; (d) nightmare; (e) OSA-related grunting; (f) RBD; (g) seizure; (h) sleep talking; (i) sleep terror; (j) snoring; (k) stridor (due to UA narrowing); and (l) wheezing.
Vocalizations during sleep	(a) Confusional arousal; (b) malingering; (c) nightmare; (d) nocturnal seizure; (e) RBD; (f) sleep talking; and (g) sleep terror.
Oral movements	(a) Facial mandibular myoclonus; (b) rhythmic movement disorder; (c) seizure; and (d) sleep bruxism.
Nighttime sensation of obstruction in upper airway or GI tract	(a) GER (± aspiration); (b) OSA; (c) panic disorder; (d) sleep-related choking syndrome; (e) sleep-related abnormal swallowing syndrome; (f) sleep-related laryngospasm; and (g) sleep terrors.
Dyspnea or choking during sleep	(a) COPD; (b) GER (± aspiration); (c) CHF (paroxysmal nocturnal dyspnea); (d) nocturnal asthma; (e) OSA; (f) panic disorder; (g) sleep-related choking syndrome; (h) sleep-related laryngospasm; and (i) sudden unexplained nocturnal death syndrome.

Nighttime eating	(a) Hypoglycemia; (b) Kleine-Levin syndrome; (c) medication induced (e.g., zolpidem and related drugs); (d) nocturnal eating syndrome; (e) OSA; (f) PUD; and (g) sleep-related eating disorder.
Cataplexy-like features	(a) Arrhythmias; (b) conversion disorder; (c) moderate-severe fatigue; (d) malingering; (e) myasthenia gravis; (f) neuromuscular weakness; (g) orthostatic hypotension; (h) periodic paralysis; (i) psychosis, (j) seizure (partial complex, atonic or absence); (k) syncope; (l) TIA; and (m) vestibular dysfunction.
Restless legs-like symptoms	(a) Akathisia related to the use of neuroleptic agents or dopamine receptor antagonists; (b) arthritis; (c) claudication; (d) habitual leg "twitching"; (e) nocturnal leg cramps; (f) peripheral neuropathy; (g) positional leg discomfort; and (h) sleep starts.

Insomnia

Insomnia is a disorder characterized by repeated difficulty with either falling or staying asleep, despite adequate opportunity, condition and time to do so. Associated with impairment of daytime function and occurs ≥ 3 nights a week and persists for ≥ 1 month. Sleep disturbance can be classified as *sleep-onset insomnia* (difficulty falling asleep), *sleep-maintenance insomnia* (frequent or prolonged awakenings), *terminal insomnia* (final morning awakening that is earlier than desired), or *nonrestorative sleep* (unrefreshed feeling upon awakening that is not due to insufficient sleep). Based on its duration, insomnia is considered *transient* if sleep disturbance lasts only a few days, *acute* if < 1 month, *subacute* if 1-3 months, or *chronic* if > 3 months. Finally, insomnia can be classified based on etiology of sleep disturbance as *primary (idiopathic) insomnia* if it is not related to any underlying medical, neurological or psychiatric disorder, or medication use, abuse or withdrawal (e.g., idiopathic insomnia, paradoxical insomnia and psychophysiologic insomnia) or *comorbid insomnia* if it is associated with a medical, neurological or psychiatric disorder, or medication use, abuse or withdrawal.

About 30-50% of adults report occasional insomnia. An estimated 6-10% of adults complain of chronic insomnia. Prevalence is greater among women, older adults, shift workers, and persons who are poor, ill, widowed or divorced.

Consequences of insomnia include increased likelihood of accidents and development of a psychiatric illness; increase in subjective sleepiness, fatigue and cognitive impairment; impaired interpersonal, academic and occupational functioning; and diminished QOL. Insomnia with *short* sleep duration is associated with increased risk of HTN, type 2 DM, cardiovascular events and all-cause mortality. Insomnia with *long* sleep duration is associated with an increase in cardiovascular and all-cause mortality.

Pathophysiologic model of insomnia

Several mechanisms may be responsible for sleep disturbance in persons with insomnia, including somatic and cognitive hyperarousal, persistent sensory perception and information processing, intrinsic sleep instability, circadian dysrhythmia, dysregulation of homeostatic sleep drive and dysfunctional cognitive processes.

Factors related to the development and maintenance of sleep disturbance can be classified into three groups (Spielman's model), namely predisposing, precipitating and perpetuating factors.

	Description	*Examples*
Predisposing factors	Increase risk of developing insomnia; present prior to the start of insomnia	(a) Decreased homeostatic sleep drive; and (b) physiologic or psychological hyperarousal.
Precipitating factors	Trigger the start of insomnia	(a) Acute illness; (b) adverse effects of medications or substances; (c) changes in sleep environment or sleep-wake schedule; and (d) stressful life events.
Perpetuating factors	Sustain the sleep disturbance	(a) Dysfunctional cognition; (b) maladaptive behaviors; (c) performance anxiety; (d) poor sleep hygiene; and (e) substance or medication use.

Specific causes of insomnia

There are several specific causes of insomnia, either a primary disorder or comorbid condition.

	Main features	*Associated features*
Adjustment insomnia	Sleep disturbance due to an identifiable acute stressor (e.g., momentous life event, change in sleeping environment or an acute illness).	Duration of insomnia is < 3 months. Sleep normalizes with resolution of the acute stressor or once the individual adapts sufficiently to the stressor.
Altitude insomnia	Sleep disturbance develops during ascent (> 2000-4000 meters) due to periodic breathing during sleep as a result of hypoxia and respiratory alkalosis.	Arousals can occur during the hyperpneic phase of periodic breathing. Symptoms resolve with acclimatization or after descent to lower altitudes.
Behavioral insomnia of childhood	Can be either *limit-setting type* (bedtime resistance due to inadequate enforcement of bedtime by caregiver), or *sleep-onset association type* (problematic associations required for sleep to occur).	*Limit-setting sleep disorder* – Repetitive stalling or refusal to go to sleep at an *appropriate* time when requested to do so. Sleep comes naturally and quickly when limits to further activities at bedtime are strictly enforced. *Sleep-onset association disorder* – Inability to fall asleep unless certain desired conditions

		(e.g., favorite toy or presence of a caregiver) are present at bedtime.
Fatal familial insomnia	Progressive sleep disturbance and insomnia, with sleep loss eventually becoming total. Other features include apathy, dysarthria, ataxia and tachycardia. Vivid dreaming and spontaneous lapses into a dreamlike state (oneiric stupor) with motor activity. Terminates in stupor, coma and death generally within 12 months to a few years after its onset.	Autosomal dominant disorder secondary to a prion disease. The hereditary form is due to a GAC to AAC mutation at codon 178 of the prion PRNP gene at chromosome 20. This cosegregates with a methionine polymorphism at codon 129. Cases of sporadic fatal insomnia do not demonstrate the mutation at codon 178 but possess the codon 129-methionine polymorphism on both alleles.
Food allergy insomnia	Sleep disturbance develops as a result of ingestion of a specific food or drink.	Other symptoms of allergy (e.g., rash or gastrointestinal discomfort) may also be present.
Idiopathic insomnia	Longstanding insomnia that is not associated with any identifiable etiology.	Onset during infancy or early childhood. Chronic life-long course without periods of remission. Increased risk of developing major depression.
Inadequate sleep	Sleep disturbance due to activities or	Examples include excessive caffeine use or

hygiene	behavior that increase arousal or decrease sleep propensity and that are under a person's control.	irregular sleep-wake schedules.
Paradoxical insomnia (sleep state misperception)	Subjective reports of chronic severe insomnia (very minimal or no sleep) during most nights associated with no PSG evidence of significant sleep disturbance. Individuals often overestimate SOL and underestimate TST compared to objective measures of sleep.	No daytime napping or impairment of daytime functioning. Chronic course.
Psychophysiologic insomnia	Chronic (≥ 1 month) sleep disturbance secondary to heightened cognitive (rumination and intrusive thoughts) and somatic (increased agitation and muscle tone) arousal at bedtime. Learned maladaptive sleep-preventing behavior. Excessive anxiety and frustration about inability to sleep.	Conditioned arousal is limited to a person's own bed and bedroom (sleep is frequently better in another room). Unlike adjustment sleep disorder, this type of insomnia persists even after resolution of the inciting stressor/s. Lastly, unlike generalized anxiety disorder (i.e., anxiety is present in several aspects of daily living), anxiety in psychophysiologic insomnia is limited to issues related to sleep.
Medical disorders that can cause insomnia	Medical disorders precipitate or exacerbate sleep disturbance.	Conditions include chronic pain syndromes, GER, CHF, nocturia, nocturnal angina and

		nocturnal asthma.
Neurological disorders that can cause insomnia	Neurological disorders precipitate or exacerbate sleep disturbance.	Conditions include dementia and PD.
Psychiatric disorders that can cause insomnia	Psychiatric disorders precipitate or exacerbate sleep disturbance.	Conditions include mood disorders, anxiety disorders, PTSD and schizophrenia.
Medications and substances that can cause insomnia	Sleep disturbance is related to use or abuse of, or withdrawal from, medications or substances.	Agents that can cause insomnia include anorexiants, antidepressants (e.g., fluoxetine or protriptyline), β-blockers, bronchodilators, decongestants, steroids, stimulants and certain substances (alcohol, caffeine and nicotine).

Evaluation of insomnia

Obtaining a comprehensive sleep, medical and social history forms the basis of any assessment of persons with complaints of insomnia.

	Description
History	Clinical history, bed partner interviews, sleep diary and validated questionnaires.
Physical examination	As needed, to assess for comorbid disorders.
Laboratory testing	As needed, to assess for comorbid disorders
Psychometric tests	As needed, to assess for comorbid disorders
Polysomnography	Not routinely indicated. May be considered for insomnia suspected to be due to SRBD, PLMD or paradoxical insomnia. General changes in sleep architecture consists of SOL $\geq$ 30 minutes, WASO $\geq$ 30 minutes, SE < 85% and TST < 6-6.5 hours. However, PSG may be normal in some patients (e.g., paradoxical insomnia or sleep disturbance due to environmental factors).
Actigraphy	Not routinely indicated. Common findings include TST < 440 minutes, SOL > 12 minutes and number of awakenings > 5.

Therapy of insomnia

Goals of insomnia therapy are alleviation of nighttime sleep disturbance and relief/elimination of daytime consequences. Approaches include general measures (e.g., sleep hygiene, addressing factors that can precipitate or perpetuate sleep disturbance, and identifying and treating comorbid causes of insomnia), non-pharmacologic therapy (cognitive behavioral treatments) and use of pharmacologic agents.

Cognitive behavioral therapies for insomnia are considered first-line treatments for chronic insomnia (both primary and comorbid). Techniques include cognitive therapy, paradoxical intention, relaxation techniques, sleep restriction and stimulus control. CBT-I is generally more effective in decreasing SOL but less effective in increasing TST compared to pharmacotherapy. Short-term benefits of CBT-I are comparable to pharmacologic therapy. Unlike pharmacotherapy, beneficial effects are sustained over time after the initial treatment period. At long-term follow-up, CBT-I is more effective than pharmacotherapy.

	Rationale	Technique
Cognitive therapy	Addresses dysfunctional beliefs (inappropriate expectations and excessive worry) accompanying insomnia.	Include *decatastrophization, cognitive restructuring, attention shifting* and *reappraisal* that identify irrational cognitive processes, challenge unrealistic concerns, and provide a more appropriate understanding of sleep disturbance and daytime impairment.
Paradoxical intention	Designed to decrease performance anxiety	Tell patient to "Go to bed at night and to try to

	associated with efforts to fall asleep.	stay awake as long as you can."
Relaxation techniques	Reduction of somatic and cognitive hyperarousal.	Progressive muscle relaxation (for somatic arousal; sequential tensing and relaxing of various muscle groups throughout the body), biofeedback (for somatic arousal) and guided imagery (for cognitive arousal).
Sleep hygiene	Encourage bedtime activities and behaviors that enhance sleep propensity. Eliminate activities and behaviors that curtail sleep propensity. A necessary component of therapy for insomnia but is rarely sufficiently effective, by itself, to reverse sleep disturbance.	Instructions include (a) maintaining a regular bedtime and waking time; (b) moderate-intensity aerobic exercise during the day; and (c) avoidance of prolonged naps during the day, spending excessive time awake in bed, ingestion of alcohol and caffeine close to bedtime, smoking close to bedtime, using medications that can cause insomnia, or engaging in stimulating activities late in the evening.
Sleep restriction	Increasing homeostatic sleep drive (due to SD) by reducing TIB. TIB is subsequently increased once SE improves.	Tell patient to "Maintain a daily sleep log. Limit time spent in bed to actual sleep time only (at least 4.5-5 hours per night). Advance or delay bedtime based on calculated SE ([TST/TIB] X

		100%) for the prior 5 nights until the desired sleep duration is reached. Advance bedtime by 15-30 minutes if SE is greater than 90%. Delay bedtime by 15-30 minutes if SE is less than 80%. Do not change bedtime if SE is between 80% and 90%. Wake up at the same time every morning. Do not nap during the day."
Stimulus control	Designed to strengthen the association of the bedroom and bedtime to a conditioned response for sleep.	Tell patient to "Use the bed only for sleep or sex. Lie down to sleep only when sleepy. If unable to fall asleep, get out of bed and go to another room. Engage in a restful activity, and return to bed only when sleepy."

Pharmacotherapy of insomnia

Hypnotic agents are indicated for transient sleep disruption, chronic primary insomnia that fails to respond to CBT-I, and chronic comorbid insomnia that does not improve with treatment of the underlying condition and CBT-I. Hypnotic agents may enhance sleep but they do not necessarily improve daytime performance. Additionally, there are minimal long-term beneficial effects on sleep following discontinuation of hypnotic agents. Ramelteon or zaleplon are recommended for sleep-onset insomnia. BZ, low-dose doxepin, eszopiclone or zolpidem may be considered for sleep-onset and sleep-maintenance insomnia. Eszopiclone, zolpidem-ER and ramelteon appear to be effective for long-term treatment of chronic insomnia. There is insufficient evidence regarding the efficacy of sedating antipsychotic agents, antihistamines and botanical compounds for the treatment of insomnia. Elimination half-lives of hypnotic agents are listed.

	Agents	*Clinical use*
< 1 hour	Ramelteon, zaleplon	Used primarily for sleep-onset insomnia.
2 to 6 hours	Eszopiclone, triazolam, zolpidem	Useful for concurrent sleep-onset-/-maintenance insomnia.
6 to 24 hours	Doxepin (low-dose), estazolam, temazepam	Useful for early morning awakenings and daytime anxiety.
> 40 hours	Flurazepam, quazepam	Useful for early morning awakenings and daytime anxiety.

Hypnotic agents for insomnia

General recommendations include (a) using the lowest effective dose; (b) administration at bedtime (hypnotic agents should ideally be taken ~ 15 minutes before desired sleep time); (c) instructions to allow sufficient time in bed (based on drug half-life) and avoidance of potentially hazardous activities after drug ingestion; (d) regular monitoring of drug efficacy and adverse effects; and (e) adjusting dose in the elderly or in persons with renal or hepatic impairment.

	Characteristics	*Notes*
Benzodiazepines	Bind to the gamma-aminobutyric acid-benzodiazepine (GABA-BZ) receptor complex. Benzodiazepines, in addition to having hypnotic properties, are also potent anxiolytics, myorelaxants and anticonvulsants. FDA-approved agents include estazolam, flurazepam, quazepam, temazepam and triazolam. These agents are approved for ≤ 35 days of use.	Adverse effects include (a) rebound daytime anxiety [with short-acting agents]; (b) daytime sleepiness [with long-acting agents]; (c) cognitive and psychomotor impairment; (d) complex sleep-related behaviors; (e) development of tolerance; (f) withdrawal symptoms; (g) dependency and abuse liability; (h) relapse; (i) rebound insomnia; and (j) respiratory depression and worsening of OSA.
Non-benzodiazepine benzodiazepine	Bind to the gamma-aminobutyric acid-benzodiazepine (GABA-BZ) receptor complex.	Compared to conventional benzodiazepines, these agents have (a)

receptor agonists	Duration of action (shortest to longest) is zaleplon < zolpidem < eszopiclone.	similar hypnotic action; (b) no muscle relaxant, anticonvulsant or anxiolytic properties; and (c) less likely to cause rebound insomnia, withdrawal symptoms or tolerance.
Melatonin receptor agonist	Selective agonist for the SCN melatonin receptor subtypes, MT1 (attenuation of arousal) and MT2 (phase shifting of circadian rhythms). Peak levels within 1 hr. Short half-life of 1-2.5 hours. Indicated for sleep-onset insomnia ($\downarrow$ SOL). Unscheduled by FDA.	No significant abuse liability, cognitive or psychomotor impairment, or rebound insomnia with drug discontinuation. No significant effects on sleep architecture. Contraindications include use of fluvoxamine and hepatic impairment.

Sedating antidepressants	Except for low-dose doxepin, sedating antidepressants are not recommended for the treatment of insomnia.	Doxepin, at low doses, acts as a H1 histamine receptor antagonist. With an estimated half-life of 15 hours, it is useful for sleep-maintenance insomnia.
Sedating antipsychotic agents	Limited published data on their appropriate use for insomnia. Not recommended for the treatment of insomnia.	Sedating antipsychotic agents include quetiapine and olanzapine. Can cause extrapyramidal symptoms, cardiac conduction abnormalities and orthostatic hypotension.
Non-prescription hypnotic agents	First generation histamine antagonists (e.g., diphenhydramine or doxylamine) constitute the majority of over-the-counter hypnotic agents.	Not recommended for the treatment of insomnia. Limited published data on their efficacy and safety as sleep aids for insomnia.
Melatonin	Used primarily for treating insomnia associated with CRSDs. Short half-life of 20-45 minutes.	Not FDA-approved for the therapy of insomnia.
Botanical compounds	Inconclusive evidence for the efficacy of kava, passionflower, skullcap or valerian as treatment for insomnia.	Hepatotoxicity has been described with kava and valerian.

Hypersomnia

Excessive sleepiness is defined as an inability to consistently achieve and sustain wakefulness and alertness to accomplish the tasks of daily living. EDS can manifest as frequent napping, sleep attacks or microsleep episodes. EDS can also present as hyperactivity in children or as automatic behavior. Causes of hypersomnia are listed.

	Essential features	Associated features
Behaviorally-induced insufficient sleep syndrome	EDS is due to chronic voluntary, but unintentional, SD. This is the most common cause of EDS.	Improvement in symptoms occurs following longer sleep duration.
Idiopathic hypersomnia	Constant sleepiness despite sufficient, or even increased, amounts of nighttime sleep and daytime napping. No identifiable cause.	Automatic behavior, confusion upon awakening (sleep inertia), disorientation, "evening" chronotype, fatigue, headaches, hypnagogic hallucinations, orthostatic hypotension, Reynaud's-type vascular symptoms, sleep paralysis and syncope.
Narcolepsy	Refer to next section	Refer to next section
Recurrent hypersomnia	Recurrent episodes of EDS that occur weeks or months apart. Normal sleep, alertness, cognitive function and general behavior	Either monosymptomatic (sleepiness only, such as menstrual-related hypersomnia) or polysymptomatic/Kleine Levin syndrome

	between episodes.	(sleepiness, hyperphagia and hypersexuality).
Hypersomnia due to medical disorders	EDS despite sufficient nighttime sleep duration (> 6 hours). Cataplexy is absent.	Includes hepatic encephalopathy, hypothyroidism, Niemann Pick type C disease, Prader-Willi syndrome and renal failure.
Hypersomnia due to neurological disorders	EDS despite sufficient nighttime sleep duration (> 6 hours). Cataplexy is absent.	Includes CNS infection, sarcoidosis or tumor, head trauma / traumatic brain injury, PD, multiple sclerosis, myotonic dystrophy and stroke.
Hypersomnia due to psychiatric disorders	EDS despite sufficient nighttime sleep duration (> 6 hours). Cataplexy is absent.	Includes atypical depression, bipolar type II mood disorder, seasonal affective disorder, schizoaffective disorder and somatoform disorders.
Hypersomnia due to drugs or substances	Use or abuse of sedative-hypnotic agents, or withdrawal from stimulant agents.	

Narcolepsy

A neurological disorder characterized by the clinical tetrad of EDS and manifestations of REM sleep physiology during wakefulness (e.g., cataplexy, sleep paralysis and sleep hallucinations). Only about 10-15% of persons with narcolepsy demonstrate this full tetrad. EDS is related to the loss of lateral and posterior hypothalamic hypocretin neurons. Clinical variants include narcolepsy without cataplexy (accounts for 10-50% of cases) and secondary narcolepsy (due to medical disorders, such as hypothalamic and brainstem lesions). Clinical features of narcolepsy are listed below.

	Essential features	*Associated features*
Excessive sleepiness	Generally, the first, primary and most disabling symptom of narcolepsy. Commonly present for > 3 months. No other identifiable cause.	Brief naps, usually lasting 10-20 minutes, occur repeatedly throughout the day. EDS transiently improves after awakening from a nap but gradually increases within 2-3 hours. May also present with repetitive microsleep episodes. *Sleep attacks* are sudden, irresistible episodes of sleepiness that occur abruptly without warning leading to sleep during inappropriate places or circumstances.
Cataplexy	Abrupt and transient episodes of muscle atonia or hypotonia during wakefulness that	Recovery is immediate and complete, but prolonged episodes may give rise to REM

	are typically precipitated by intense emotion (e.g., laughter [most common], anger or excitement). Cataplexy is the only pathognomonic symptom of narcolepsy.	sleep. Respiratory and oculomotor muscles are spared. Memory and consciousness are unaffected. Physical examination during an episode of cataplexy may demonstrate muscle flaccidity, reduction or absence of deep tendon reflexes, and a positive Babinski sign.
Sleep hallucinations	Hallucinatory phenomena can be visual, auditory, tactile or kinetic. May be accompanied by sleep paralysis. Last a few seconds or minutes.	Occur during wakefulness at sleep onset (*hypnagogic*) or upon awakening (*hypnopompic*).
Sleep paralysis	Affects voluntary muscles with sparing of respiratory, oculomotor and sphincter muscles. Frequently accompanied by hallucinations, dyspnea and fear. Sensorium is unaffected. Duration of a few seconds or minutes. Recovery is immediate and complete.	Occur either at sleep onset (*hypnagogic*) or upon awakening (*hypnopompic*).
Sleep disturbance	Poor sleep quality with repetitive arousals and awakenings.	Affected persons may complain of sleep-maintenance insomnia.

Other clinical features	Memory impairment, automatic behavior, visual changes (blurred vision, diplopia and ptosis) and sleep inertia/drunkenness (confusion and diminished alertness immediately after waking).	Hyperactivity and learning disability (in children). Behavioral problems.
Associated disorders	Increased risk of developing SRBD (OSA and CSA), parasomnias (sleep terrors and sleepwalking), PLMS and RBD. Consider a diagnosis of narcolepsy in cases of pediatric RBD. An estimated 1/4 of persons with narcolepsy have concurrent OSA.	Increased risk of developing depression and type 2 DM.

Evaluation of hypersomnia

Chronically insufficient sleep duration or irregular sleep-wake schedules should be excluded. Subjective scales of sleepiness may not always correlate with objective measures of hypersomnia.

	Features
Clinical history and physical examination	Sleep history, sleep diary ± actigraphy and physical examination. Narcolepsy with cataplexy can be diagnosed by history alone – i.e., EDS ≥ 3 months plus cataplexy. Neurological examination is usually normal for narcolepsy and idiopathic hypersomnia.
Sleepiness scales	Subjective measures of sleepiness, such as ESS or Stanford sleepiness scale.
Polysomnography	PSG followed by MSLT is indicated to exclude narcolepsy when cataplexy is absent, atypical or equivocal. Also indicated to rule out OSA and PLMD. Monitoring esophageal pressure to exclude UARS is recommended. PSG features of narcolepsy consist of (a) ↓ SOL [< 10 minutes]; (b) SOREMP [REM SL ≤ 10-15 minutes] in 25-50% of cases; (c) ↑ N1; (d) ↑ WASO; (e) ↓/= TST; and (f) normal R. PSG features of idiopathic hypersomnia consist of ↓ SOL, ↑ SE, ↑/= TST, ↓ WASO, ↑ N3 (in some) and no change in REM SL.
Multiple sleep latency test	Sleepiness is defined by a mean SOL < 8 minutes. Mean sleep latencies (± SD) are 10 ± 4 minutes in healthy persons; 3 ± 3 minutes for narcolepsy; and 6 ± 3 minutes for idiopathic hypersomnia. ≥ 2 SOREMPs in narcolepsy. < 2 SOREMPs in idiopathic hypersomnia.
Maintenance of	May be used to monitor treatment response to stimulant medications used for EDS.

wakefulness test	
Actigraphy	Assists in excluding insufficient sleep syndrome or CRSDs.
CSF hypocretin test	CSF hypocretin-1 level ≤ 110 pg/mL or < 1/3 of mean normal control values (in the absence of severe brain pathology) in narcolepsy with cataplexy. Normal CSF hypocretin-1 levels in idiopathic hypersomnia.
HLA typing	Limited diagnostic utility and is not indicated for the diagnosis of any cause of hypersomnia.
Other tests	Performance vigilance testing. Imaging may be considered for suspected secondary narcolepsy. Medical, neurological and psychiatric assessments to exclude other disorders associated with EDS.

Therapy of hypersomnia

Treatment should be individualized. Periodically assess response to therapy.

	Features
General measures	Adequate nocturnal sleep duration. Sleep extension (for insufficient sleep syndrome). Optimal sleep hygiene. Regular sleep-wake schedules. Therapy of other concurrent sleep disorders that can cause EDS. Avoidance of potentially dangerous activities (e.g., driving) until EDS is adequately managed.
Scheduled napping	Useful for patients with narcolepsy but is seldom sufficient as sole therapy for EDS. Should not be used as a substitute to obtaining adequate nighttime sleep.
Light therapy	May be useful for SWD and JL.
Stimulant therapy	Includes caffeine, amphetamines, methylphenidate or modafinil/armodafinil. Stimulant therapy improves, but does not always completely reverse, EDS due to narcolepsy. Avoid chronic use to replace obtaining sufficient sleep duration.
Hypnotic agents or sodium oxybate	Treatment of sleep disturbance (in narcolepsy).
REM sleep suppressant agents or sodium oxybate	Treatment of cataplexy, sleep paralysis and sleep hallucinations (in narcolepsy).

Obstructive sleep apnea

Repetitive reduction (hypopnea) or cessation (apnea) of airflow, despite the presence of respiratory efforts, due to partial (hypopnea) or complete (apnea) UA occlusion during sleep. OSA can be classified based on severity as *mild* (AHI 5-15 events per hour), *moderate* (16-30) or *severe* (> 30).

Compared to controls, persons with OSA tend to have narrower UA that are more vulnerable to collapse. The most common sites of UA obstruction are the retropalatal (behind the palate) and retrolingual (behind the tongue) regions. Repetitive UA obstruction due to reduced activity of UA dilating muscles during sleep is associated with snoring (alternating with periods of silence); episodic falls in SaO_2; arrhythmias (relative bradycardia during airway obstruction followed by tachycardia during termination of apnea); arousal at the termination of the event; and ↑ BP in the immediate post-apneic period.

Risk factors for OSA include (a) + family history of OSA; (b) male gender [for adults]; (c) menopausal state in women; (d) aging; (e) excess body weight; (f) specific cranio-facial and oropharyngeal features [neck circumference > 17 inches in men and > 16 inches in women], brachycephaly, nasal narrowing or congestion, macroglossia, low-lying soft palate, enlarged tonsils and adenoids, mid-face hypoplasia, retrognathia and micrognathia; (g) hereditary syndromes [Crouzon, Down, Pierre-Robin and Treacher Collins]; (h) race; (i) smoking and alcohol use; (j) certain medications [muscle relaxants, sedatives, anesthetics and opioid analgesics]; and (k) specific primary disorders [acromegaly, androgen therapy and polycystic ovarian syndrome).

Features of obstructive sleep apnea

OSA is a systemic disorder; this is underscored by its diverse clinical features, physical examination findings and associated conditions.

Common clinical features

(a) EDS; (b) ADHD [in children]; (c) changes in mood [particularly treatment-resistant depression]; (d) decline in performance at work or school; (e) dry mouth/throat sensation upon awakening; (f) fatigue; (g) GER; (h) impaired cognition; (i) morning headaches; (j) nighttime diaphoresis; (k) nocturia; (l) nonrestorative or unrefreshing sleep or naps; (m) repeated awakenings with gasping or choking; (n) snoring; and (o) witnessed apneas.

Common physical findings

(a) Crowded posterior pharyngeal space; (b) dental malocclusion; (c) enlarged tonsils and adenoids; (d) excess body weight; (e) high, narrow hard palate; (f) large neck circumference; (g) large uvula; (h) low-lying soft palate; (i) macroglossia; (j) narrow oropharynx; (k) nasal septal deviation or turbinate hypertrophy; and (l) retro- or micrognathia. Physical examination may be entirely unremarkable.

Common associated conditions

(a) Cardiac arrhythmias; (b) CHF; (c) insomnia; (d) insulin resistance; (e) ischemic heart disease; (f) nocturnal seizures; (g) parasomnias; (h) pulmonary HTN and cor pulmonale; (i) sleep bruxism; and (j) systemic HTN.

Consequences of obstructive sleep apnea

There is great individual variability in OSA's impact on different organ systems. Some of these differences can be explained by disease severity or duration, presence of comorbid disorders, or genetic susceptibility.

	Description
General	Greater mortality (among young and middle-age adults).
Respiratory variables	Decrease in SaO_2 and PaO_2, and increase in $PaCO_2$ during sleep.
Cardiovascular variables	Increased systemic and pulmonary artery pressure. Reduced LV and RV output. Higher PVR.
Sleep quality	Sleep disturbance with greater number of arousals.
Neurocognitive and psychiatric effects	Depression and anxiety; reduced QOL, alertness and vigilance; and impairment of neurocognitive performance (executive function, learning and memory).
Systemic hypertension	Increase in both systolic and diastolic BP as well as failure of systemic BP to fall during sleep ("non-dipping"). Due, at least in part, to greater sympathetic nervous system activity. Increase in renin-angiotensin activity and sodium retention may also contribute.
Pulmonary hypertension and cor pulmonale	Prevalence of pulmonary HTN in OSA without cardiopulmonary disease is about 20%. Greater likelihood in persons with daytime hypoxemia and hypercapnia, morbid obesity or underlying COPD. Degree of pulmonary HTN is generally mild.
Coronary artery disease	Nocturnal angina. Change in usual timing of sudden cardiac death from 6 AM-12 PM in the

	general population to 12 AM-6 AM. Due to systemic inflammation, endothelial dysfunction, metabolic derangements, vasomotor imbalance and coagulation abnormalities.
Congestive heart failure	Greater prevalence of OSA in persons with CHF. OSA, in turn, may worsen heart function (can cause both systolic and diastolic dysfunction).
Cardiac arrhythmias	Sinus arrhythmia [most common], atrioventricular block, bradycardia, premature ventricular contractions, complex ventricular ectopy, sinus pause or arrest, and non-sustained ventricular tachycardia. Increased incidence, and recurrence following cardioversion, of atrial fibrillation.
Cerebrovascular disease	Bidirectional relationship – increased risk of strokes in persons with OSA and increased risk of OSA following strokes.
Metabolic dysfunction	Higher risk of insulin resistance, altered glucose metabolism and type 2 DM. Increased serum leptin levels [but low leptin activity due to leptin resistance] and ghrelin levels.
Miscellaneous	(a) Accidents; (b) erectile dysfunction; (c) GER; (d) nocturia; and (e) parasomnias.

Evaluation of obstructive sleep apnea

Sleep testing, either using PSG or PSAT, is indicated for the diagnosis of OSA.

	Description
Clinical history	Most clinical screening tests, because of false negative rates, miss a significant proportion of persons with OSA.
Physical examination	High Mallampati score (i.e., only uvula and soft palate, or only hard palate visible).
Laboratory testing	Routine screening for hypothyroidism is *not* indicated unless other clinical features suggestive of hypothyroidism are present.
PSG and/or PSAT	Required for the diagnosis of OSA. The current standard of practice is a laboratory study with technologist-attended PAP titration using either full-night (with separate diagnostic and PAP titration studies) or split-night (consisting of an initial diagnostic portion and a subsequent PAP titration on the same night) protocols. PSAT should only be performed as part of a comprehensive sleep evaluation. PSAT may be considered in persons with high pre-test probability of OSA; full PSG should be performed if results are negative or non-diagnostic in persons with high clinical suspicion of OSA.
MSLT	Indicated if EDS persists during optimal PAP therapy.
Upper airway imaging studies	May be considered for patients with craniofacial syndromes, especially prior to surgical therapy. Includes lateral cephalometric views, CT or MRI of the UA.

Therapy of obstructive sleep apnea

PAP therapy is the treatment of choice for most patients with OSA. Weight management is important for obese persons.

	Description
General measures	Sleep hygiene. Avoidance of alcohol, BZ, opioids and muscle relaxants that can decrease UA dilator muscle activity. Safety counseling (i.e., avoidance of driving whenever drowsy).
Optimal weight management	Should be combined with primary treatment for OSA. Consider closely monitored very low energy diet or bariatric surgery for morbidly obese persons. Regular exercise.
Positional therapy	Avoidance of a supine sleep position in persons whose respiratory events occur exclusively or predominantly during supine sleep and in whom PSG demonstrates a normal AHI in the lateral or prone sleep position. Techniques include placing tennis balls in a pocket sewn in the back of a pajama top, use of positional vests or belts, use of wedge pillows, or positional alarms.
Oxygen therapy	Not indicated as sole therapy for OSA. It may be considered for persons with significant nocturnal hypoxemia that is not controlled by PAP therapy alone.
Nasal dilators	Not sufficiently effective when used alone to treat OSA.
Pharmacologic treatments	Topical nasal corticosteroids may be a useful adjunct to primary therapies for OSA in persons with concurrent rhinitis. Modafinil/armodafinil is recommended for treating residual EDS in persons on effective PAP therapy and with no other known cause of EDS.
Positive airway pressure	Optimal PAP setting should eliminate all apneas, hypopneas, snoring and respiratory event-

therapy	related arousals in all sleep positions and in all stages of sleep. Indicated for (a) AHI of ≥ 15 events per hour; or (b) AHI of ≥ 5 and ≤ 14 events per hour *plus* complaints of EDS, impaired cognition, mood disorder or insomnia, *or* documented HTN or CAD, *or* history of stroke.
Oral devices for OSA	Indicated for (a) snoring; (b) mild to moderate OSA; and (c) severe OSA [in some]. Include mandibular repositioners, which displace the mandible and tongue anteriorly; and tongue-retaining devices, which secure the tip of the tongue in a soft bulb located anterior to the teeth to hold the tongue in an anterior position. Reported efficacy from 50-80%. Compliance is about 50-90%. Follow-up PSG/PSAT after optimal fit has been achieved is recommended to assure therapeutic efficacy as are periodic assessments by a dentist and sleep physician.
Upper airway surgery for OSA	Indicated primary for persons with definitive craniofacial or UA abnormalities responsible for OSA. PSG/PSAT following UA surgery is recommended to determine its therapeutic efficacy. Long-term follow-up is required. Tonsillectomy and adenoidectomy may be considered in childhood OSA due to adenotonsillar enlargement. Other procedures include (a) nasal surgeries *to increase dimensions of nasal airway*; (b) uvulopalatopharyngoplasty *to increase dimensions of retropalatal airway*; (c) laser midline glossectomy with lingualplasty, tongue base reduction with hyoepiglottoplasty, genioglossal advancement, hyoid myotomy and suspension, or mandibular advancement *to increase dimensions of retrolingual airway*; (d) uvulopalatopharyngoglossoplasty and maxillo-mandibular advancement *to increase dimensions of retrolingual, retropalatal and transpalatal airway*; and (e) tracheotomy *to bypass upper*

airway.

Novel therapies for OSA	Transnasal insufflation (continuous high-flow, warm-humidified air is administered via an open nasal cannula); oropharyngeal exercises (can reduce AHI and improve both EDS and sleep quality); nasal expiratory resistance device; oral pressure therapy; and hypoglossal nerve stimulation.
Management of residual sleepiness during PAP therapy	Assure optimal PAP pressure and adherence. Distinguish EDS from fatigue. Identify and manage other disorders that can give rise to EDS (e.g., insufficient sleep, narcolepsy or mood disorder). Eliminate (if possible) use of sedating medications. Modafinil or armodafinil may be considered as adjunct therapy for improving alertness and wakefulness. Neither drug reverses the negative impact of OSA on cardiovascular morbidity. It should *not* be used to replace PAP therapy for OSA.

Positive airway pressure modalities

PAP therapy acts like a pneumatic splint that maintains UA patency during sleep.

	Features
Continuous positive airway pressure (CPAP)	A single constant pressure is provided throughout the respiratory cycle.
CPAP with expiratory pressure relief technology (CFlex)	A single pressure is provided but allows for a transient reduction in pressure during expiration and a subsequent return of pressure to baseline setting before initiation of the next inspiration. Pressure relief is adjustable (setting of 1-3) and is proportional to expiratory flow (i.e., greater relief in the setting of more expiratory effort).
Bi-level positive airway pressure (BPAP)	Two independent pressure levels are provided during the respiratory cycle, namely a higher level during inspiration (inspiratory positive airway pressure [IPAP]) and a lower pressure during expiration (expiratory positive airway pressure [EPAP]). BPAP with expiratory pressure relief technology (Biflex) is also available. BPAP can be used in one of 3 modes, namely spontaneous setting (all breaths are initiated by the patient), spontaneous-timed setting (breaths are triggered by the device if spontaneous breaths fall below a predetermined rate), or timed rate (a fixed number of breaths per minute are triggered by the device).
Auto-titrating positive airway pressure (APAP)	Variable pressures are provided to respond to changes in UA resistance or airflow using device-specific diagnostic and therapeutic algorithms. Automatically and continuously adjusts the

	delivered PAP to maintain UA patency. P95 (pressure exceeded only 5% of the time) and P90 (pressure exceeded only 10% of the time) are often used to determine a fixed CPAP setting. Both P95 and P90 can be affected by poor compliance, mask leaks or inadequate (i.e., too low) pressure range settings.
Adaptive servo ventilation (ASV)	Provides constant ventilation based on either peak flow or minute ventilation measurements. Automatically adjusts settings in response to specific respiratory events, such as (a) increased positive end-expiratory pressure for obstructive events; (b) increased inspiratory pressure support for hypopneas; (c) decreased inspiratory pressure support for hyperpneas/hyperventilation; and (d) back up rate for impending apneas. Thus, pressure support (difference between EPAP and IPAP) increases during periods of hypoventilation and decreases during periods of hyperventilation.
Average volume assured pressure support (AVAPS)	Bi-level with average volume assured pressure support that maintains a stable tidal volume.
Non-invasive positive pressure ventilation (NIPPV)	Two pressure levels are provided at a set rate to assist ventilation. May be considered for persistent sleep-related hypoventilation and CO_2 retention that persist during PAP and O_2 therapy.

Benefits and consequences of PAP therapy

PAP therapy is associated with a number of beneficial effects. Unfortunately, it can also lead to several unwanted consequences.

Beneficial effects of PAP therapy for OSA	*Adverse consequences of PAP therapy for OSA*
(a) Reduced mortality; (b) less EDS; (c) better sleep quality; (d) decrease in AHI; (d) improved SaO_2; (e) better QOL and mood; (f) enhanced neurocognitive function [inconsistent data]; (g) improved mood; (h) better BP control; (i) improvements in heart function in persons with CHF; (j) reduced pulmonary artery pressures in persons with pulmonary HTN; (k) decreased prevalence of atrial and ventricular arrhythmias, and less recurrence of atrial fibrillation after cardioversion); (l) reduced systemic pro-inflammatory mediators and oxidative stress markers; (m) improved insulin sensitivity; (n) improvement of GH, testosterone, leptin and ghrelin levels; and (o) decreased healthcare utilization.	(a) Aerophagia and gastric distention; (b) arousals; (c) barotrauma [e.g., pneumothorax, pneumomediastinum and pneumocephalus]; (d) changes in certain craniofacial measurements; (e) chest discomfort and tightness; (f) claustrophobia; (g) eye irritation [conjunctivitis]; (h) facial skin irritation, rash or abrasion; (i) mask and mouth leaks; (j) nasal congestion, dryness, epistaxis or rhinorrhea; (k) noise from the device; (l) sensation of suffocation or difficulty with exhalation; and (m) sinus discomfort or pain.

Adherence to PAP therapy

PAP use should be monitored objectively. Objective compliance (use for > 4 hours per night for 70% of nights) ranges from 50-80%. Average nightly use is about 5 hours. Intermittent PAP use is common. Patterns of adherence to PAP therapy can often be discerned within the first few days of starting therapy.

Common reasons for non-adherence to PAP therapy	Factors predicting better adherence to PAP therapy	Effective approaches to improve PAP adherence
(a) Difficulty with exhaling against high expiratory pressures [consider Cflex or BPAP therapy]; (b) excessively high pressures [consider trial of APAP or BPAP therapy, or adjunctive therapy with sleep position treatment or oral devices]; and (c) gastric distention due to aerophagia [consider BPAP therapy].	(a) High AHI; (b) severe EDS; (c) self-referral for medical care; and (d) positive patient attitudes and self-efficacy.	(a) Patient education; (b) heated humidification [inconsistent data]; and (c) one-time use of long-acting NBBRA during the CPAP titration night.

Central sleep apnea

Repetitive cessation of airflow during sleep due to reduction or loss of ventilatory effort. Can give rise to sleep fragmentation, insomnia or EDS. Persons with CSA may also be asymptomatic.

PSG is necessary for the diagnosis of CSA. PSG features consists of (a) cessation of respiration and ventilatory effort lasting ≥ 10 seconds; (b) absence of chest and abdominal movement in RIP or strain gauge; (c) no respiratory muscle activity in diaphragmatic EMG; (d) no changes in pressure in esophageal pressure monitoring; and (e) rounded profile in nasal pressure monitoring. Diagnostic criteria are ≥ 5 central apneas per hour of sleep; in persons with both obstructive and central events, central apneas/hypopneas should constitute > 50% of the total respiratory events. Major differences between obstructive and central apneas are listed.

	Obstructive apneas	*Central apneas*
Oxygen desaturation	More severe	Less severe
Hemodynamic changes	Greater	Less
Respiratory effort	Present	Absent
Snoring	More prominent	Less prominent

Classification of central sleep apnea

Causes of CSA can be classified based on level of ventilation as either hypercapnic or non-hypercapnic.

	Description and mechanisms	Causes
Hypercapnic	Hypoventilation during sleep (high sleep $PaCO_2$). Often associated with daytime hypoventilation (high waking $PaCO_2$). Due to decreased ventilatory response to hypercapnia.	(a) Central alveolar hypoventilation; (b) neuromuscular disorders; and (c) chronic use of long-acting opioids.
Non-hypercapnic	Not associated with daytime hypoventilation (normal or low waking $PaCO_2$). Mechanisms include increased ventilatory response to hypercapnia (as $PaCO_2$ levels increase during sleep, brief arousals trigger a hyperventilatory "overshoot" that lowers $PaCO_2$ below its apneic threshold and gives rise to central apneas) and episodic hypoxemia (leading to increase in minute ventilation, reduction in CO_2 and, eventually, central apnea).	(a) Idiopathic CSA; (b) sleep-onset or post-arousal CSA; (c) CSA due to CHF; (d) high altitude periodic breathing; and (e) complex sleep apnea.

Causes of central sleep apnea

CSA can be *primary* (idiopathic) or *secondary* to other medical disorders (more common than the primary form). Causes of secondary CSA are cardiac, renal and neurological disorders (e.g., CHF, renal failure, brainstem lesions, head injury, neuromuscular disorders, stroke and autonomic dysfunction), and chronic use of long-acting opioids.

	Description
Primary CSA	Unknown etiology. Related to increased ventilatory response to hypercapnia leading to fall in $PaCO_2$. Rare condition.
Cheyne Stokes respiration	Periodic breathing with recurring episodes of crescendo-decrescendo ventilation separated by central apneas or hypopneas. Central apneas are post-hyperventilatory in nature. There is also a corresponding waxing-waning pattern of SaO_2. Prevalence of 25-40% in CHF, and 10% in stroke. Also seen in persons with renal failure. In CHF, CSR cycle time (> 45 seconds; typically 60-90 seconds) is directly proportional to circulation time and inversely related to LVEF.
High altitude periodic breathing	Cycles of central apnea and hyperpnea developing on ascent to high altitude (usually > 4,000-7,600 meters). > 5 CAs per hour of sleep. Risk factors include (a) greater hypoxic ventilatory drive, (b) higher elevation, (c) faster speed of ascent, and (d) male gender.
CSA due to medication use	Dose-dependent depression of hypercapnic (and, in some, hypoxic) respiratory drive, with CAs, periodic respiration, bradypnea, Biot breathing or prolonged

	hypoventilation, related to chronic use ($\geq$ 2 months) of long-acting opioids (e.g., methadone).
CSA due to CHF	CSA and CSR can develop in persons with CHF. Prevalence and severity are correlated with LV function. CSA is present in about 1/3 of persons with CHF.
Sleep-onset central apnea	Central apneas may develop if $PaCO_2$ (higher during sleep and lower during wakefulness) fluctuates above or below the apnea threshold. Generally transient and resolves as sleep progresses. Repetitive sleep-onset central apneas can give rise to sleep-initiation insomnia.
CSA during PAP titration	Development or increasing frequency of CSA or CSR during application of CPAP in persons with predominantly obstructive or mixed apneas during the initial diagnostic study. Also referred to as complex sleep apnea or PAP treatment-emergent CAs. Risk factors for complex sleep apnea are underlying CHF or CAD, male gender, and presence of central or mixed apneas during the diagnostic study.

Therapy of central sleep apnea

Treatment of non-hypercapnic CSA generally differs from that of hypercapnic CSA.

	Description
General	Treatment of underlying causes (e.g., CHF). Reassurance for sleep onset CAs. Avoidance of respiratory depressants (e.g., BZ or opioid narcotics) in hypercapnic CSA.
Oxygen therapy	May benefit some persons with non-hypercapnic CSA (e.g., CSR or complex sleep apnea). Indicated for high-altitude periodic breathing.
Inhaled CO_2	Inhaled CO_2 or addition of dead space. Indications are not well established.
Pharmacologic therapy	Consists of acetazolamide (for high-altitude periodic breathing and CSA/CSR in CHF); theophylline (for CSA or CSR related to CHF, and for CSA related to prematurity in newborns); medroxyprogesterone (for OHS) and hypnotic agents (for sleep-onset central apneas and possibly for idiopathic CSA).
Positive airway pressure therapy	CPAP or BPAP for CSA/CSR due to CHF; CPAP, BPAP or ASV for complex sleep apnea; and BPAP with back-up rate or AVAPS for sleep apnea/hypoventilation.
NIPPV	For persons with hypercapnic CSA.
Other therapies	Cardiac resynchronization therapy and transplantation in selected patients with end-stage CHF.

Hypoventilation syndromes

The main feature is elevated $PaCO_2$ during sleep (either > 45 mmHg, or < 45 mmHg but is abnormally increased relative to waking levels). Commonly accompanied by sleep-related O_2 desaturation. Waking ABG may be normal or abnormal. Mechanisms include decrease in minute ventilation, abnormal V/Q relationships or sleep-related reductions in ventilatory chemosensitivity and respiratory load responsiveness. PSG features consist of SaO_2 during sleep < 90% for > 5 minutes with a nadir ≥ 85%; > 30% of TST with SaO_2 < 90%; and ↑ $PaCO_2$. Therapy includes treatment of underlying disorder/s, ventilatory assistance during sleep (BPAP, AVAPS or NIPPV), and, in some patients, a trial of respiratory stimulants.

	Description
Idiopathic alveolar hypoventilation	Not secondary to a respiratory, chest wall or neuromuscular disorder. Normal respiratory mechanics. Believed to be due to decreased chemoresponsiveness to CO_2.
Congenital central alveolar hypoventilation syndrome	Failure of automatic control of breathing results in hypoxemia and hypercapnia during sleep. Waking and voluntary respiration are relatively normal. Due to reduced responsiveness of central and peripheral chemoreceptors to O_2 and CO_2. Onset of hypoventilation usually in infancy and may present as respiratory failure, cyanosis, ALTE or cor pulmonale. Hypoventilation is worse during sleep than wakefulness, and is more severe during N3 than REM sleep. Associated features include autonomic dysfunction, Hirschsprung disease and neural crest tumors. Many cases involve *de novo* mutations of the PHOX2B gene.

Obesity hypoventilation syndrome	Development of hypoxemia (SaO_2 < 90%) and hypercapnia ($PaCO_2$ > 45 mmHg [wake], and > 10 mmHg increase in $PaCO_2$ compared to wake values [sleep] in obese (BMI > 30 kg/m2) persons. Other features include polycythemia, pulmonary HTN and OSA. About 10% of persons with OSA have OHS. About 90% of persons with OHS have OSA. No other known causes of hypoventilation.
Medical and neurological disorders causing alveolar hypoventilation	Can arise from respiratory disorders (interstitial lung disease, pulmonary HTN, lower airways obstruction or chest wall disorders), or neurological disorders (amyotrophic lateral sclerosis, diaphragm paralysis, myopathy, post polio syndrome, spinal cord injury or brainstem stroke).

Parasomnias

Parasomnias are physical or experiential phenomena that occur during the sleep period. They manifest as activation of skeletal muscles or autonomic nervous system during sleep. Disorders of arousal, occurring predominantly during N3 sleep, consist of confusional arousal, sleep terror and sleepwalking. Parasomnias that generally occur during REM sleep include nightmares, RBD and isolated sleep paralysis. Therapy consists of (a) sleep hygiene; (b) avoidance of precipitating factors; (c) trial of scheduled awakenings [patients are awakened about 15-30 minutes before the time when parasomnia typically occurs and then allowed to return to sleep]; (d) environmental precautions; and (e) clonazepam or melatonin for RBD.

	Clinical features	Associated features	Evaluation and treatment
Catathrenia	Intermittent expiratory groaning or moaning during sleep (predominantly REM sleep) following episodes of bradypnea.	Hoarseness on waking and mild daytime fatigue. No associated respiratory distress, emotional anguish, abnormal motor activity, O_2 desaturation or cardiac arrhythmias.	Normal neurological and UA examination. Normal sleep architecture during PSG. Therapy consists of trial of PAP or mandibular repositioner devices.
Confusional arousal	Episodes of confusion following spontaneous or forced arousals from sleep. Main clinical features consist of disorientation, inappropriate	Events can be precipitated by SD, alcohol use, fever, forced awakenings, idiopathic hypersomnia, medications (CNS depressants), narcolepsy, OSA,	Therapy may consist of avoidance of SD, trial of sleep extension, trial of scheduled awakenings, psychotherapy (for marked psychological distress)

	behavior, amnesia and inconsolability. Minimal or no signs of fear or autonomic hyperactivity.	PLMD, shift work, sleep terrors and sleepwalking.	and possibly off-label use of TCA and BZ.
Exploding head syndrome	Awakening with a loud sound or sensation of explosion in the head. May be a variant of sleep start.	Not associated with pain or neurological complications. Can give rise to insomnia.	
Isolated sleep paralysis	Persistence of REM-sleep muscle atonia during wakefulness. Accompanied by hallucinations in 25-75% of cases.	Respiration is unaffected and consciousness is preserved.	
Nightmare disorder	Unpleasant and frightening dreams that often abruptly awaken the sleeper. Typically occur during REM sleep in the 2nd half of the nocturnal sleep period.	Full alertness and good recall of preceding dream on awakening. Delayed return to sleep. Minimal autonomic changes (no significant tachycardia or tachypnea). Frequent nightmares can lead to insomnia, EDS and anxiety.	Therapy consists of (a) reassurance; (b) sleep hygiene; (c) cognitive behavioral therapy [e.g., image rehearsal]; (d) psychotherapy; (e) trial of REM sleep suppressants for severe cases; and (f) prazosin or neuroleptic agents in PTSD-

			related nightmares.
REM sleep behavior disorder	Abnormal "dream enacting" behavior and complex motor activity during REM sleep associated with loss of REM-related muscle atonia or hypotonia. Rapid awakening and full alertness. Good dream recall. ANS activation is uncommon.	Predisposing factors include α-synucleopathies, aging, alcohol withdrawal, caffeine use, male gender, medications (e.g., TCA, SSRI, SNRI, MAOI, biperiden and cholinergic agents), olivopontocerebellar atrophy, and stroke. Chronic and progressive course. Complications include injuries to self or bed partner, and sleep fragmentation.	Evaluation should include comprehensive neurological testing for any underlying α-synucleinopathic neurodegenerative disorder. PSG with additional EMG monitoring of the upper extremities [flexor digitorum] and time-synchronized video recording is indicated for diagnosis. PSG features include increased muscle tone or phasic EMG activity during REM sleep. Therapy consists of (a) avoidance of known precipitants; (b) low-dose clonazepam at bedtime; (c) melatonin; and (d) environmental precautions in

			the bedroom.
Sleep enuresis	Recurrent involuntary voiding during sleep that occurs ≥ twice a week after 5 years of age.	Classified as primary or secondary: *primary* if a child has never been consistently dry during sleep for 6 consecutive months; or *secondary* if a child or adult who had previously been dry for 6 consecutive months and then begins bedwetting ≥ twice a week for a period of ≥ 3 months.	Spontaneous cure rate of primary sleep enuresis is 15% annually. Evaluation commonly consists of a urinalysis and urine culture. Urologic evaluation is indicated for suspected structural urinary tract disorders. Treatment of enuresis includes bell and pad therapy (70% effective), bladder training or pharmacotherapy (desmopressin or imipramine).
Sleep-related dissociative disorder	Nocturnal fugue state that develops within several minutes after an awakening.	Defensive, self-mutilating, sexualized or violent behavior; vocalization or ambulation; and amnesia.	

Sleep-related eating disorder	Repetitive bouts of involuntary eating or drinking during arousals from sleep. Arousals appear to be triggered by learned behavior rather than by real hunger or thirst.	Lack of, or partial, awareness of the abnormal behavior; total or partial amnesia; and consumption of high-caloric foods, inappropriate substances or inedible material.	Should be differentiated from *nocturnal eating syndrome*, which occurs at night with the patient awake, is accompanied by full recall of the event, and is not associated with consumption of inappropriate food items. Treatment consists of behavioral therapy.
Sleep terror	Abrupt awakening with profound fear and intense autonomic discharge (tachycardia, tachypnea, sweating and mydriasis). Awakenings generally occur during N3 sleep, often in the 1st third of the night.	Vocalization (talking or screaming), ambulation, confusion and amnesia.	Therapy consists of (a) avoidance of SD; (b) trial of sleep extension; (c) behavioral therapy; (d) trial of scheduled awakening; (e) trial of low-dose BZ; (f) hypnosis; and (g) stress management.
Sleepwalking	Automatic, semi-purposeful behavior, including ambulation, during the sleep period. Most	Confusion, amnesia for the episode, inappropriate behavior (may give rise to violent activity)	Spontaneous resolution of childhood cases usually by puberty. Treatment consists of

frequently occurs in stage N3 sleep, during the 1st half of the night.	and diminished arousability.	anticipatory scheduled awakening; medications, such as BZ or TCAs (when cases are frequent or associated with injuries); hypnosis; environmental precautions; and avoidance of precipitating factors.

Restless legs syndrome

Restless legs syndrome is a neurological disorder characterized by an urge to move, or unpleasant sensations, involving the legs (and less commonly the arms) that (a) begin or worsen during periods of rest or inactivity; (b) are relieved transiently by movement; and (c) are worse, or occur only, at night. Among children (2-12 years of age), diagnosis requires either presence of all 4 adult criteria *and* description of leg discomfort in the child's own words; or presence of all 4 adult criteria *and* ≥ 2 of the following: sleep disturbance, RLS in parent or sibling, or PLMI of ≥ 5 per hour.

RLS has a prevalence of 3-15% in the general population. About 70-90% of persons have PLMS. Conversely, one-third of persons with PLMS have RLS. Most common in middle-aged and older adults, but onset can occur at any age. Course is chronic, and remission is more likely in mild (vs. more severe) and in secondary (vs. primary) RLS.

Pathophysiology most likely involves dysregulation of dopaminergic system (↓ dopamine receptor binding, presynaptic dopaminergic hypofunction and ↓ tyrosine hydroxylase in substantia nigra). Abnormal iron metabolism may be contributory (↓ brain iron in putamen, red nucleus and substantia nigra on brain MRI; ↓ CSF ferritin; ↑ CSF transferrin; ↓ serum ferritin; and impaired iron uptake and transport across the blood-brain barrier). Ferritin is a cofactor for tyrosine hydroxylase, the rate-limiting enzyme for dopamine synthesis, and iron deficiency is thought to reduce the number of dopamine receptor binding sites.

Classification of restless legs syndrome

RLS is classified, based on etiology, into *primary* (idiopathic) or *secondary*. Primary cases may be related to abnormalities in dopaminergic systems. RLS can also be classified based on age of onset into *early* or *late* onset.

	Primary RLS	Secondary RLS
Age of onset	Early or late	Generally late
Family history	More likely	Less likely
Severity of symptoms	Milder	More severe
Progression of symptoms	Less rapid	More rapid
Reversibility	Less likely	More likely

	Early onset	Late onset
Age of onset	≤ 35-45 years	> 45 years
Etiology	Mainly primary (idiopathic)	May be primary (idiopathic) or secondary
Progression	Slower	More rapid

Risk factors and consequences of restless legs syndrome

The table below lists the risk factors and consequences of RLS.

Risk factors	Consequences
(a) ADHD; (b) aging; (c) alcohol or caffeine ingestion; (d) Charcot-Marie-Tooth disease type 2; (e) COPD; (f) DM; (g) family history; (h) female gender (among adults); (i) fibromyalgia; (j) gastric surgery; (k) iron deficiency anemia [↓ serum ferritin levels]; (l) medication use [SSRI, SNRI, TCA, MAOI, lithium, antihistamines, neuroleptics, dopamine antagonists, antiemetics, antipsychotic agents, calcium channel blockers, and some anticonvulsant drugs]; (m) mood disorder; (n) multiple sclerosis; (o) narcolepsy; (p) PD; (q) peripheral neuropathy; (r) peripheral venous disease; (s) pregnancy; (t) rheumatoid arthritis; (u) SD; (v) smoking; (w) spinal stenosis or lumbosacral radiculopathy; (x) stroke; (y) thyroid disease; and (z) uremia.	(a) Cognitive impairment; (b) depressed mood; (c) EDS due to sleep fragmentation; (d) HTN; (e) impaired glucose metabolism (in some); (f) ↓ QOL; and (g) sleep-onset and sleep-maintenance insomnia.

Evaluation of restless legs syndrome

Differential diagnoses of RLS include akathisia related to the use of neuroleptic agents or dopamine receptor antagonists, arthritis, claudication, habitual leg "twitching", nocturnal leg cramps, peripheral neuropathy, positional leg discomfort and sleep starts.

	Description
Routine evaluation	Clinical history, family history and physical examination.
Neurological examination	Normal in primary RLS.
Laboratory evaluation	CBC, serum iron, ferritin, folate, electrolytes, thyroid function tests, fasting glucose and renal panel.
Polysomnography	Not routinely indicated, but may be considered if sleep disruption persists despite control of RLS. PSG features include low sleep input pattern and sleep instability (cyclic alternating pattern). PLMW > 15 per hour may be present prior to sleep onset. PLMS may be present.
Suggested immobilization test	PSG is performed for 1 hour prior to habitual evening bedtime with the patient awake, sitted upright in bed and with legs outstretched. PLMW > 40 per hour supports the diagnosis of RLS.

Therapy of restless legs syndrome

Dopaminergic medications are the first-line agents for treating RLS.

	Description
General measures	Sleep hygiene. Treatment of underlying causes or precipitating factors.
Nonpharmacologic therapy	Includes counter stimulation (e.g., warm baths, massage or pneumatic compression devices), light-to-moderate daytime exercise, stretching and relaxation techniques.
Iron supplementation	Consider if serum ferritin < 50 ng/mL.
Dopaminergic agent	Includes levodopa, pergolide, pramipexole, ropinirole and rotigotine. Decreases RLS symptoms and frequency of PLMS, and improves sleep quality. Dopaminergic agents are not recommended for use in children and pregnant women.
Benzodiazepine	Includes clonazepam. Reduces RLS symptoms and PLMS-related arousals, and improves sleep quality.
Opioid agent	Includes codeine, oxycodone and propoxyphene. Decreases RLS symptoms and PLMS. May be considered for severe symptoms refractory to other therapy.
Anticonvulsant agent	Includes carbamazepine, gabapentin and pregabalin. Gabapentin may be considered for RLS accompanied by pain.
Other medications	Includes clonidine, amantadine and selegiline.

Periodic limb movements during sleep

Recurrent leg movements during sleep that commonly consist of partial flexion of the ankle (dorsiflexion), knee and hip, and extension of the big toe. Involvement of the upper extremity consists of flexion at the elbow. Can also occur while sitting or lying during restful wakefulness, referred to as periodic limb movements during wakefulness (PLMW). Share many of the risk factors of RLS. Disorders that are associated with PLMS include RLS (most important), narcolepsy, RBD, OSA and spinal cord injury. PSG is required for diagnosing PLMS (using EMG of the anterior tibialis muscles). Periodic limb movement index (PLMI) is the total number of PLMS per hour of TST. PLMI is abnormal if (1) > 5 in children and (2) > 15 in adults.

Periodic limb movement disorder (PLMD) is defined as symptomatic PLMS with complaints of sleep disturbance or EDS. Therapy of PLMD is similar to that of RLS. Specific therapy is not indicated for asymptomatic PLMS.

Circadian rhythm sleep disorders

Caused by a recurrent or persistent misalignment between the desired or imposed sleep schedule and the circadian sleep-wake rhythm. Can be associated with insomnia or EDS (or both). CRSDs can arise from either (a) temporary misalignment between biological and environmental time (e.g., shift work disorder or jet lag), (b) abnormal circadian phase (e.g., advanced or delayed sleep phase syndromes), or (c) insufficient or absence of entrainment (e.g., irregular sleep-wake rhythm or free-running disorder). CRSDs can be classified as intrinsic (ASPS, DSPS, FRD and ISWR) or extrinsic (JL and SWD) syndromes.

	Advanced sleep phase syndrome	*Delayed sleep phase syndrome*	*Free-running (non-entrained, non-24-hour sleep-wake) circadian disorder*	*Irregular sleep-wake rhythm*
Key features	Habitually early bedtime (6-9 PM) and early wake time (2-5 AM). Major sleep period occurs *earlier* than desired or conventional bed times. Sleep, itself, is	Habitually late bedtime (1-6 AM) and late wake time (10 AM to 2 PM). Major sleep period occurs *later* than desired or conventional bed times. Sleep, itself, is	Progressive daily delay in sleep-onset and wake times. The major sleep period progressively "marches" throughout the day, afternoon and evening.	Variable, inconsistent and multiple sleep and wake periods throughout the day and night, that differ from one day to another (≥ 3 sleep episodes in a 24-hr

				period).
Main symptoms	Excessive sleepiness in the late afternoon or early evening. Morning awakenings are earlier than desired.	Sleep-onset insomnia and morning sleepiness when sleep is attempted at more conventional bedtimes.	*Periodically recurring* problems of insomnia or EDS alternating with complete, but brief, disappearance of symptoms.	Insomnia or EDS.
Demographics	Onset is commonly during middle age. Prevalence of 1% in middle-aged and older adults.	Onset is often during adolescence. Prevalence of 0.1-0.2% in the general population. More common among adolescents and young adults.	Most affected persons are totally blind and lack photic entrainment. May also affect sighted persons with dementia or mental retardation.	Rare condition. Most frequently seen in association with neurological disorders (e.g., autism, dementia or mental retardation).
Pathophysiology	Shorter than normal endogenous circadian rhythm period; overly dominant phase advance capability;	Phase delay of the circadian sleep-wake rhythm coupled with an inability to phase advance in order to	Abnormal synchronization between the endogenous sleep-wake circadian	Weak zeitgebers, poor sleep hygiene or underlying medical disorders.

	inability to phase delay; or altered homeostatic regulation of sleep.	correct the disturbance.	rhythm and the 24-hour environmental light-dark cycle.	
Evaluation	History, sleep logs or actigraphy. Phase advances in CTmin and DLMO. "Morning type" on the Horne-Ostberg test.	History, sleep logs or actigraphy. Phase delays in the timing of CTmin and DLMO. "Evening type" on the Horne-Ostberg test.	History, sleep diary or actigraphy. Progressive delays in CTmin and DLMO. A neurological evaluation to exclude any CNS pathology is recommended for sighted persons with FRD.	History, sleep logs or actigraphy.
Polysomnography	Normal if performed during the preferred advanced sleep time. ↓ SOL, ↓ TST and ↓ REM SL if performed during a conventional	Normal if performed during the habitually delayed sleep period. ↑ SOL and ↓ TST if performed during a conventional earlier	Progressively longer SOL and shorter TST when PSG is recorded at a fixed period over several days.	

	later sleep time.	sleep time.		
Differential diagnoses	Use of short-acting hypnotic agent or use of alcohol at bedtime, REM-related OSA, nightmare disorder and depression.	Psychophysiologic insomnia, idiopathic insomnia, mood and anxiety disorders, and poor sleep hygiene.	Severe DSPS.	Poor sleep hygiene and very irregular work schedules.
Therapy	Early evening bright light therapy and early morning light restriction.	Early morning light exposure and evening avoidance of light. Chronotherapy with progressive phase delay, progressive phase advancement or scheduled shift of the major sleep episode until the desired bedtime is reached. Evening melatonin.	Evening melatonin. Morning bright light therapy for sighted persons or blind persons with light perception. Maintenance of regular schedules of sleep and waking.	Evening melatonin. Daytime light exposure and nighttime light restriction. Maintenance of regular schedules of sleep and waking.

	Jet lag	*Shift work disorder*
Key features	Transient insomnia and/or EDS within 1-2 days following rapid eastward or westward air travel across multiple (≥ 2) time zones.	Sleep disturbance is directly related to non-standard work schedules.
Main symptoms	Sleep-onset insomnia and difficulty awakening the next day following eastward flights. Early evening sleepiness and early morning awakening after westward flights. Other symptoms include fatigue and malaise, gastrointestinal disturbances, decreased mood and impaired performance. Symptoms remit spontaneously within approximately a day for every time zone change.	Sleepiness and decreased alertness during night shifts; insomnia during daytime sleep periods; non-restorative sleep; and distress and functional impairment. Other complaints include chronic fatigue and malaise; cognitive decline; poor work performance; work-related accidents; absenteeism and decreased job satisfaction.
Demographics		About 20% of the workforce in industrialized countries is involved in some form of non-standard work schedule, and about 10% of shift workers develop SWD.
Pathophysiology	Lack of synchrony to the new local time zone. Individuals traveling westward are	Recurrent or persistent disparity between the timing of work and the requirement for sleep.

Therapy	Timed bright light therapy. Short-acting hypnotic agents or melatonin at bedtime for insomnia. Consider short-term use of stimulants (including caffeine) for severe cases.	Measures that increase nighttime alertness include appropriately timed bright light exposure in the workplace; napping before, or during, night work; and administration of
Differential diagnoses	Another diagnosis (e.g., psychophysiologic insomnia) should be considered if sleep disturbance persists for > 2 weeks following air travel.	Poor sleep hygiene and irregular sleep wake rhythm.
Polysomnography	↑ SE and ↓ WASO; delayed SOL with eastbound travel.	Low sleep input pattern.
Evaluation		Evaluation includes sleep diaries recorded over several days. Actigraphy may aid diagnosis. PSG is not routinely indicated.
	phase-advanced relative to the new clock time, whereas those traveling eastward are phase-delayed. North-south travel does not lead to jet lag.	Time cues of sunlight and social activities are out-of-phase with the altered sleep time. Lastly, many shift workers revert back to a traditional daytime routine during non-work days, which prevents stable synchronization between exogenous and endogenous rhythms.

	of EDS.	psychostimulants [e.g., caffeine, modafinil or armodafinil] during evening work hours. Daytime sleep can be enhanced by hypnotics, including melatonin prior to post-shift daytime sleep; and restricted daytime light exposure, such as using dark sunglasses, during the morning trip home from work.

Therapy of circadian rhythm sleep disorders

Most effective treatments for CRSDs are timed phototherapy and melatonin administration. Light therapy should be complemented by appropriate light restriction at either the start or end of the sleep period.

	Useful for
Planned napping	SWD
Phototherapy	DSPS, ASPS, FRD (for intact light perception), ISWR, SWD, JL
Melatonin	DSPS, FRD, ISWR, SWD, JL
Stimulants and hypnotics	SWD, JL

Medical, neurologic and psychiatric disorders

The relationship between sleep and medical disorders is bidirectional - sleep quality is affected by medical disorders and by medications, and vice versa.

	Clinical features	Sleep-related complaints	Changes in sleep architecture
Acromegaly	Due to excessive levels of growth hormone (usually secondary to a pituitary adenoma).	OSA and CSA are common.	
Addison disease	Low levels of cortisol.	Fatigue and sleep disruption.	
Alcohol abstinence		Sleep disturbance, including insomnia, can persist for several years.	↑ SOL, ↓ TST, ↑ WASO and ↓ N3.
Alcohol-dependent sleep disorder	Habitual use of alcohol prior to anticipated bedtime only for its sedative effects. No other patterns of behavior compatible with overt		

	alcoholism are present.		
Alcoholism		Increase in nightmares, vivid dreams, enuresis, RLS, sleep terrors, sleepwalking, snoring and OSA.	↓ SOL, ↓ WASO, ↑ N3, ↑ REM SL and ↓ R during the first part of the sleep period; and ↑ WASO, ↓ N3 and ↑ R during the second part of the sleep period.
Alcohol withdrawal, acute		Vivid, disturbing dreams, insomnia and frequent awakenings.	↑ SOL, ↑ WASO, ↓ TST, ↓ N3, ↓ REM SL and ↑ R.
Allergic disorder		Insomnia. Allergic rhinitis can increase UA resistance and exacerbate OSA.	

Alternating leg muscle activation	Brief activity of the anterior tibialis muscle of one leg that alternates with activity of the same muscle in the other leg.	Can occur with or without arousals.	Repetitive, alternating activation of the anterior tibialis EMG. Each EMG activation lasts between 0.1-0.5 seconds, ≥ 4 muscle activations occurring in sequence lasting from 1-30 seconds, and with < 2 seconds between activations.
Amyotrophic lateral sclerosis	Motor neuron disease.	EDS, insomnia, OSA, CSA, hypoventilation and nocturnal O_2 desaturation.	
Anxiety disorder, acute stress disorder	Excessive anxiety developing within 4 weeks of a traumatic experience. Medications used to treat psychiatric disorders may also cause significant sleep disturbance.	Insomnia.	Low sleep input pattern.

Anxiety disorder, generalized	Excessive anxiety or worry of ≥ 6 months duration. Medications used to treat psychiatric disorders may also cause significant sleep disturbance.	Insomnia, frequent nighttime awakenings, recurring anxiety dreams or EDS.	Low sleep input pattern, ↓ N3 and ↓ R.
Arrhythmia, cardiac	Decreased prevalence of PVCs during sleep (due to greater parasympathetic tone), and increased prevalence of ventricular arrhythmias during arousals from sleep.	Untreated OSA is associated with (a) increased incidence and recurrence of AF; and (b) increased incidence of non-sustained ventricular tachycardia and complex ventricular ectopy.	In OSA, HR slows at the onset of the apneic episode and increases after the termination of the event.
Asperger disorder	Impairment in social interaction with limited patterns of activities and interests.	Insomnia.	
Asthma	Episodic dyspnea, wheezing or coughing due to reversible	Insomnia, sleep fragmentation, EDS and nocturnal hypoxemia.	Low sleep input pattern.

	bronchoconstriction and airway hyperreactivity to specific and nonspecific stimuli.		
Atopic dermatitis		Sleep disturbance (due to frequent scratching), insomnia or EDS.	Low sleep input pattern.
Attention deficit hyperactivity disorder	Some symptoms of inattention and hyperactivity are present prior to 7 years of age, leading to impairments at home, school or work.	Variable sleep-wake schedules, sleep-onset insomnia (bedtime resistance), problematic night waking, sleep fragmentation and EDS. Increased prevalence of SRBD and PLMD.	Low sleep input pattern.
Autistic disorder	Impaired functioning in language, social interaction, behavior or interests beginning before 3 years of age.	May be associated with (a) rhythmic movement disorders (e.g., head banging) continuing beyond 10 years of age, (b)	

		insomnia, including problematic night waking, and (c) CRSD (DSPS or ISWP).	
Benign epilepsy of childhood with centrotemporal spikes (BECTS)	Hemifacial perioral numbness and focal clonic twitching of the face, tongue and mouth. Drooling and dysarthria. Preserved consciousness.	Benign clinical course. Seizures occur predominantly or exclusively during sleep.	EEG shows centrotemporal spike and sharp waves. PSG features (during nights when seizures occur): Low sleep input pattern, ↓ N3, ↑ REM SL and ↓ R.
Benign sleep myoclonus of infancy	Repetitive, brief and bilateral myoclonic jerks (involving large muscle groups, such as the trunk, limbs, or even the entire body) occurring only during sleep (predominantly during quiet sleep).	Not accompanied by seizure activity or arousals.	Myoclonus occurs as 4-5 jerks per second, recurring every 3-15 minutes.
Bipolar mood disorder	Can either be *bipolar 1* (≥ 1 manic, hypomanic or mixed episodes ± major depressive	EDS during depressive phase. Sleeplessness during manic phase. Nightmares.	Low sleep input pattern and ↓ N3. ↑ TST and ↓ REM

			SL during depressive phase. ↓ TST during manic phase. PSG abnormalities may persist even after clinical remission.
	episode) or *bipolar 2* (≥ 1 major depressive episodes plus ≥ 1 hypomanic episode, without manic or mixed episodes). Medications used to treat psychiatric disorders may also cause significant sleep disturbance.		
Blindness		Insomnia, problematic night waking and EDS. FRD in blind persons with no light perception.	↓ TST.
Brain injury (traumatic)	Risk factors for sleep disturbance include presence of skull fracture, need for surgery, and prolonged coma (> 24 hours).	*Insomnia* after injury to basal forebrain and anterior hypothalamus. *EDS* following injury to midbrain and posterior hypothalamus. Injury to brainstem respiratory neurons can give rise to	↓ TST, ↑ SOL, ↓ N3, ↓ R immediately after brain injury; and ↑ TST, ↓ SOL, ↑ N3, ↑ R after 2-4 weeks post-injury.

		OSA. *Secondary narcolepsy* after injury to lateral hypothalamus. Sleep-related *seizures* and post-traumatic *hypersomnia*.	
Cerebral degenerative disorder	Abnormalities in cognition, behavior and movement.	Persons with olivopontocerebellar degeneration may present with CSA, nocturnal stridor, OSA or RBD.	Low sleep input pattern. Muscle contractions are most prominent during N1 and N2 sleep.
Cerebral palsy		Increased risk of OSA.	
Chronic obstructive pulmonary disease	Progressive, not fully reversible, airflow limitation resulting from injury to the small airways and alveoli from noxious particles or gases. Includes emphysema and chronic bronchitis.	Repetitive awakenings, insomnia, non-restorative sleep, OSA, RLS, EDS or fatigue. Nocturnal hypoxemia and hypercapnia may develop in moderate to severe disease. "Overlap syndrome" refers	Low sleep input pattern, but may be normal. Sleep-associated O_2 desaturation that is worse during REM sleep.

		to the presence of both COPD and OSA.	
Chronic paroxysmal hemicrania	Severe unilateral, brief headaches (e.g., temporal, orbital or supraorbital) that are responsive to therapy with indomethacin.	Headaches occur during both sleep and waking. Most commonly associated with REM sleep.	Low sleep input pattern.
Cluster headache	Excruciating, unilateral (periorbital or temporal) headaches that occur in "clusters". During cluster periods, 1-3 headache attacks can occur daily, often at the same hour each day.	Headaches occur during both sleep (especially during REM sleep) and waking.	Low sleep input pattern.
Congestive heart failure	LV systolic dysfunction is an independent risk factor for OSA; conversely, OSA may contribute to worsening LV dysfunction.	Increased prevalence of OSA (1/3 of patients) and CSA/CSR (> 1/3 of patients).	CSR occurs predominantly during N1 and N2 sleep.

	Unclear if CSA/CSR independently increases risk of progression of heart failure.		
Continuous spike waves during NREM sleep	Formerly referred to as electrical status epilepticus of sleep. Associated with neurocognitive and motor impairment.	Seizures occur predominantly or exclusively during sleep. Nocturnal seizures may result in sleep disruption, EDS and insomnia. May present with or without any visible movements or clinical complaints.	Continuous and diffuse slow spike-wave complexes occur throughout NREM sleep. Discharges decrease during REM sleep and disappear with awakening. Low sleep input pattern, ↓ N3, ↑ REM SL and ↓ R during nights when seizures occur.
Coronary artery disease		Risk of CAD is increased in middle-aged persons with OSA (independent of age, BMI, BP and smoking), and is reduced by reversal of OSA.	

Cushing disease	Excess of adrenocorticosteroid hormones.	Insomnia, fatigue and OSA.	
Cystic fibrosis	Abnormal sodium and chloride transport across the epithelium results in bronchiectasis, exocrine pancreatic insufficiency, intestinal and urogenital dysfunction, and abnormal sweat gland function.	Sleep fragmentation, nocturnal coughing and sleep-related hypoxemia.	
Dementia	Significant, and often progressive, neurocognitive impairment. Includes tauopathies (Alzheimer, corticobasal degeneration and progressive supranuclear palsy) and α-synucleinopathies (diffuse Lewy body dementia,	Tauopathies are commonly associated with insomnia, CRSDs and SRBDs. α-synucleinopathies are associated with insomnia, SRBDs, RBD and EDS. CRSDs include irregular sleep-wake rhythm and/or reversal of day-night circadian	Low sleep input pattern. ↓ Sleep spindles and K-complexes. ↓ N3. ↑ REM SL and ↓ R (especially in advanced disease).

	multiple system atrophy and PD).	rhythmicity. Nocturnal confusion, agitation and wandering ("sun downing"). Increased risk for RBD in persons who have dementia with Lewy bodies.	
Depression, atypical	Lethargy, increase in appetite, weight gain and sensitivity to rejection. Medications used to treat psychiatric disorders may also cause significant sleep disturbance.	EDS.	↑ TST and ↓ REM SL. PSG abnormalities may persist even after clinical remission.
Depression, major	≥ 1 major depressive episode without any manic, hypomanic or mixed episodes. Medications used to treat psychiatric disorders may also cause significant sleep disturbance.	Insomnia or EDS/fatigue. Insomnia may persist following remission of depression.	Low sleep input pattern. ↓ N3 (particularly during the 1st NREM period), ↓ REM SL and ↑ REM density. ↓ N3 and ↓ REM SL may persist during clinical remission.

Diaphragm paralysis		Nocturnal hypoxemia (worse during REM sleep) and SRBD.	
Down syndrome		Increased risk of EDS, OSA, CSA, insomnia, PLMD, bruxism and sleep talking.	
Duchenne muscular dystrophy		Sleep disturbance, insomnia, EDS, OSA, CSA and nocturnal hypoxia.	Low sleep input pattern and $\downarrow$ R.
Dysmenorrhea	Painful uterine cramps occurring during menses.	Deceased sleep quality and EDS.	$\downarrow$ SE.
Eating disorder		Insomnia and repetitive nighttime awakenings.	
Endometriosis	Presence of endometrial tissue outside the uterus (e.g., abdomen or pelvis).	Sleep disturbance secondary to pain.	
Environmental sleep disorder	Sleep complaints that are directly due to adverse environmental factors, such	Insomnia, EDS or parasomnia.	Low sleep input pattern if PSG is performed in the usual sleep environment.

	as excessive noise.		Normal sleep architecture and sleep duration if PSG is performed in the sleep laboratory where home-related environmental disturbances are absent.
Fibromyalgia	Fatigue and multiple tender areas throughout the body.	Nonrestorative sleep.	Low sleep input pattern and ↓ N3. Alpha EEG activity may be present during NREM sleep (alpha-NREM EEG sleep).
Fragmentary myoclonus	Episodes of asynchronous and asymmetric twitch-like contractions of the muscles of the face, trunk and extremities that last from 10 minutes to over an hour.	Generally asymptomatic but can give rise to sleep disturbance and EDS.	> 5 brief EMG discharges per minute. No EEG abnormalities.
Functional bowel disorders	Chronic gastrointestinal symptoms are not associated with significant	Poor sleep quality, frequent awakenings, nighttime abdominal discomfort and	PSG is generally normal.

	anatomical, metabolic or infectious abnormalities. Include functional dyspepsia and irritable bowel syndrome.	nonrestorative sleep.	
Gastroesophageal reflux	Backflow of gastric acid and other gastric contents into the esophagus due to incompetent barriers at the gastroesophageal junction.	Sleep fragmentation, insomnia, EDS, nocturnal heartburn, dyspnea, coughing, choking, retrosternal chest pain or a bitter or sour taste.	Repeated arousals followed by swallowing (i.e., increase in chin EMG activity) and ↓ N3. Arousals are associated with episodic reductions in distal esophageal pH.
Generalized tonic-clonic seizures on awakening	Seizures that occur predominantly or exclusively during sleep.	Sleep disruption, EDS and insomnia.	PSG features (during nights when seizures occur): Low sleep input pattern, ↓ N3, ↑ REM SL and ↓ R.
Human immunodeficiency virus (HIV) infection	Risk factors for sleep disturbance include duration of disease, presence of HIV-	Insomnia, sleep fragmentation and EDS. Possible ↑ risk of OSA.	↓ SOL, ↓ SE, ↑ WASO, ↓ N2 and ↑ N3 (↓ N3 in terminal stages).

	related symptoms, T-cytotoxic/suppressor cell counts and antiviral therapy.	Efavirenz administration can give rise to insomnia, frequent awakenings and vivid dreams.	
Hypertension	OSA is a risk factor for HTN.	Loss of nocturnal fall in BP ("dipping" phenomenon) in OSA.	
Hypnagogic foot tremor	Rhythmic tremors of the feet or toes that occur during the wake-sleep transition or during stages N1 or N2 sleep.	Can result in sleep-onset insomnia or sleep disruption if severe.	Recurrent trains of 1-2 Hz leg or foot EMG potentials lasting 10-15 seconds.
Hypnic headache	Generalized or unilateral headaches that occur during sleep and may be accompanied by nausea.	Headaches occur only during sleep (most commonly during REM sleep and less commonly during N3 sleep).	Low sleep input pattern.
Hypnotic-dependent sleep disorder	Sleep disturbance related to habitual use of hypnotic agents.	Development of insomnia during abrupt drug withdrawal.	

		Residual EDS following use of long-acting hypnotic medications.	
Hypothyroidism		EDS, OSA and CSA. Hypothyroidism is *not* a significant and independent predictor of OSA.	
Infectious mononucleosis		EDS.	↓ SOL and ↑ TST.
Juvenile myoclonic epilepsy	Consists of three seizure types: (a) myoclonic jerks, (b) generalized tonic-clonic seizures [occasionally] and (c) absence seizures.	Bilateral massive myoclonic jerks affecting the limbs occur on awakening. Generalized tonic-clonic seizures can occur during sleep or on awakening.	Symmetric and synchronous 4-6 Hz EEG polyspike and wave discharges.
Juvenile rheumatoid arthritis		EDS. Greater likelihood of OSA, RLS and PLMD.	Low sleep input pattern.
Lennox-Gastaut syndrome	Seizure syndrome with intellectual and personality changes.		Generalized fast EEG rhythms during sleep.

Long sleeper	Sleep time is substantially longer than typical for the person's age group (i.e., > 10 hours for a young adult).	EDS develops if TST is less than the required amount of sleep.	Normal SE and ↑ TST. MSLT is normal following usual amount of nighttime sleep.
Lyme disease	Multisystem (rheumatologic, neurological and dermatologic) disease caused by *Borrelia burgdorferi*.	EDS, insomnia, frequent awakenings, RLS and nocturnal leg jerking. Sleep disturbances can persist for several years.	↑ SOL, ↓ SE and ↑ WASO. Alpha waves may intrude into NREM sleep.
Meningomyelocele		Increased risk of UA obstruction and OSA. Central apneas and hypoventilation can develop in cases associated with type II Arnold-Chiari malformation.	
Mental retardation	Sub-average intellectual functioning.	Insomnia, sleep fragmentation, PLMS and rhythmic movement disorder.	

Migraine headache	Episodic headaches, often unilateral, associated with nausea, vomiting, photophobia or phonophobia.	Headaches occur during both sleep and waking. Commonly have their onset during sleep. Can occur during N3 or REM sleep.	Low sleep input pattern.
Morvan's fibrillary chorea	Autoimmune disease characterized by neuromyotonia (abnormal muscular twitching and cramping that occurs at rest and exacerbated by exercise), weakness, delirium, excessive sweating and pruritus.	Insomnia (including agrypnia excitata or severe total insomnia of long duration), ↓ duration of sleep, oneiric confusion and abnormal REM sleep.	↓ sleep spindles and K complexes. REM sleep without atonia.
Multiple sclerosis	Destruction of myelin sheath causes progressive neurodegenerative disease (blurred vision, loss of balance, numbness, tingling	Insomnia, SRBD (OSA, CSA, respiratory arrest or episodic hyperventilation), RBD, RLS, PLMD and secondary narcolepsy.	

	and weakness).		
Multiple system atrophy	Characterized by parkinsonism, ataxia and autonomic dysfunction.	RBD and SRBD. Sudden death during sleep may occur due to bilateral vocal cord abductor paralysis.	Laryngoscopy during sleep aids in diagnosis of vocal cord paralysis. Management, in many cases, consists of tracheotomy. CPAP may be considered in persons unwilling to undergo tracheostomy.
Myasthenia gravis	Due to post-synaptic cholinergic receptor autoantibodies.	OSA and CSA. Nocturnal O_2 desaturation (predominantly during REM sleep) can develop.	
Myotonic dystrophy	Myotonia and muscle wasting secondary to a trinucleotide repeat disorder.	EDS, insomnia, sleep disruption, OSA, CSA, hypnagogic hallucinations, and hypoventilation (especially during REM sleep).	Low sleep input pattern.

Nocturnal frontal lobe epilepsy	Dystonic-dyskinetic, choreoathetoid or ballistic posturing and semi-purposeful activity occurring repeatedly during NREM sleep (nocturnal paroxysmal dystonia). Clonic or tonic-clonic activity.	EDS and/or insomnia. Abnormal and complex motor behavior (e.g., sleep terrors, sleepwalking, bicycling or pelvic thrusting). Sleep fragmentation and frequent arousals. Vocalization and automatisms.	Diagnosis requires a comprehensive history and an expanded EEG montage. Video-PSG may aid diagnosis. Spike and slow wave EEG complexes in some, but may have no evident abnormal ictal or interictal discharges. PSG features (during nights when seizures occur) include low sleep input pattern, ↓ N3 and REM, and ↑ REM SL.
Nocturnal temporal lobe epilepsy	Motionless staring and automatisms (e.g., lip smacking) are common.	Sleep disruption and EDS. Insomnia. Impaired consciousness and post-ictal confusion.	Diagnosis requires a comprehensive history and an expanded EEG montage. Video-PSG may aid diagnosis.

Obsessive-compulsive disorder	Presence of persistent intrusive and irrational thoughts (obsessions) and their related behaviors (compulsions).	Insomnia.	Low sleep input pattern and ↓ REM SL.
Pain syndrome		Sleep fragmentation, EDS and fatigue.	Low sleep input pattern.
Panic disorder	Attacks of extreme anxiety or fear that begin spontaneously and without any identifiable precipitating factor. Medications used to treat psychiatric disorders may also cause significant sleep disturbance.	Abrupt awakenings with immediate and sustained wakefulness and good recall of the event. Delayed return to sleep. Insomnia. Fears of going to sleep.	PSG may be normal, or may demonstrate ↑ SOL and ↓ SE in some.
Parkinson disease	Clinical triad of muscle rigidity, brady/hypokinesia and resting tremors.	Sleep-related complaints are common, including insomnia, sleep fragmentation, EDS, fatigue,	Low sleep input pattern and ↓ R.

		parasomnias (RBD, nightmares, sleepwalking and hallucinations), RLS, PLMD, CRSDs (reversal of circadian day-night rhythms), SRBD (CSA, OSA and hypoventilation), nocturia and painful leg cramps.	
Peptic ulcer disease	Patients with PUD have greater gastric acid secretion during sleep compared to normal healthy individuals.	Repeated arousals and awakenings, and nocturnal abdominal pain (onset is commonly within the 1st 4 hours of sleep).	
Personality disorder	Chronic patterns of cognition, behavior and interpersonal relationships that deviate from usual societal expectations.		Low sleep input pattern and ↓ REM SL in borderline disorder.

Poliomyelitis and post polio syndrome	Poliomyelitis is a lower motor neuron disease. Post polio syndrome is characterized by new progressive muscle atrophy, weakness and pain affecting respiratory, bulbar or extremity muscles that develops following poliomyelitis.	EDS, SRBD and nocturnal hypoventilation.	Low sleep input pattern.
Polycystic ovarian syndrome	Increased ovarian production of male sex hormones. Irregular or absent menstrual cycles, infertility, weight gain, insulin resistance and hirsutism.	Increased risk for OSA.	
Post-traumatic stress disorder	Chronic hyperarousal and anxiety associated with preoccupation and	Insomnia. EDS. Re-experiencing of the original traumatic event through	Low sleep input pattern and ↓ R.

	repetitive re-experiencing (e.g., flashbacks) of a severely traumatic or life-threatening event.	frequent anxiety dreams, sleep terrors and nightmares. Bedtime resistance (in children).	
Pre-eclampsia	Characterized by hypertension, proteinuria, pedal edema and headaches.	Higher prevalence of EDS, snoring, OSA and PLMS.	↑ WASO.
Premenstrual dysphoric disorder	Fatigue, mood changes and daytime impairment developing prior to menses.	Insomnia or EDS.	↓ SE, ↑ N2 and ↓ R; but may be unremarkable.
Premenstrual syndrome	Abdominal bloating, greater irritability and increased fatigue occurring prior to menses. Symptoms remit with menses.	Insomnia, frequent awakenings, non-restorative sleep, unpleasant dreams, nightmares and EDS.	No significant changes in sleep architecture.
Progressive supranuclear		Insomnia, OSA and nocturia.	↑ Phasic twitching during

palsy			REM sleep. ↓ REM sleep. Absence of vertical eye movements during REM sleep.
Propriospinal myoclonus at sleep onset	Spontaneous muscle jerks that occur during the transition from wake to sleep and that disappear at sleep onset.	Myoclonus starts in the abdominal and truncal muscles and spread slowly rostrally and caudally.	
REM sleep-related sinus arrest	Recurrent episodes of sinus arrest, with periods of asystole lasting up to 9 seconds in duration, occurring during REM sleep.	Most patients are asymptomatic (palpitations or vague chest pain may occasionally be present). Episodes are not associated with arousals or SRBD.	Daytime ECG and coronary angiography are generally normal.
Renal disease, end-stage	Sleep disturbance can develop in about 60-80% of patients with ESRD.	EDS, insomnia or reversal of day-night sleep patterns. High prevalence of OSA, RLS and PLMD.	Low sleep input pattern. ↑ N1, ↑ N2, ↓ N3 and ↓ R.

Restrictive lung disease	Reduced lung volumes due to disorders involving the lung parenchyma, pleura or chest wall. Include kyphoscoliosis, interstitial lung disease and severe obesity.	Sleep disturbance, frequent awakenings, non-restorative sleep, insomnia, EDS, SRBD (OSA and CSA) and nocturnal O_2 desaturation (transient or sustained). Obesity is associated with snoring, OSA, OHS and nocturnal hypoventilation.	Low sleep input pattern.
Rett syndrome	Multiple neurological deficits (psychomotor retardation, language impairment, gait disturbance, deceleration of head growth and abnormal hand movements, such as hand wringing) that develop following a period of apparently normal prenatal and perinatal (1st 5 months)	Insomnia and problematic night wakings (children).	Low sleep input pattern.

	development.		
Rhythmic movement disorder	Repetitive, stereotypic and rhythmic movements generally occurring during sleep onset and light sleep. If frequent, can give rise to sleep-onset insomnia. Includes head banging, head rolling, body rolling and body rocking.	No seizure activity.	0.5-2 movements per second lasting < 15 minutes. Frequency of movements: N1 > N2/N3 > R. No seizure activity.
Schizophrenia	Chronic psychiatric disorder characterized by hallucinations, delusions, disorganized speech, affective flattening, limited goal-directed behavior, and restricted thought and speech production.	Insomnia, EDS, frightening dreams, polyphasic sleep periods and reversal of day-night sleep patterns. Insomnia is common during acute psychotic decompensation, when a person may remain awake for prolonged periods. EDS can develop during (a)	Low sleep input pattern, ↓ N3 and ↓ REM SL. ↓ REM rebound after SD. ↓ TST and ↓ R during the waxing phase of the disorder. Normalize during the waning, post-psychotic and remission phases of the disorder. ↑ REM SL with successful

		the waning phase of schizophrenia or (b) residual schizophrenia.	therapy of schizophrenia.
Seasonal affective disorder	Development of depressive episodes during the fall and winter. Depression is absent during spring and summer, when some persons may experience hypomanic symptoms.	EDS and ↑ sleep requirements in the fall and winter. Decreased sleep requirements (in some) during spring and summer.	
Short sleeper	Habitual sleep duration of ≤ 5 hours daily despite voluntary attempts to lengthen sleep duration.	Normal sleep onset, quality, continuity and consolidation. No impairment in daytime functioning.	↓ SOL and ↓ TST. Normal MSLT.

Sleep hyperhidrosis	Profuse sweating that occurs during sleep. May be related to OSA, febrile illness, pregnancy or menopause.	Can lead to frequent awakenings and sleep fragmentation.	
Sleeping sickness	Human African trypanosomiasis caused by *Trypanosoma brucei* gambiense or rhodesiense. Transmitted by the bite of an infected tsetse fly.	EDS, insomnia (not uncommon) and reversal of sleep-wake periods.	Few vertex sharp waves, sleep spindles and K complexes. ↓ REM SL (SOREMPs).
Sleep-related abnormal swallowing syndrome	Pooling of saliva in the oral cavity during sleep due to abnormal swallowing mechanisms.	Arousals from sleep due to coughing and choking. A "gurgling" sound can be heard preceding each coughing spell.	
Sleep-related bruxism	Repetitive teeth grinding or jaw clenching during sleep.	Episodes may be associated with arousals.	Overall sleep architecture is normal. Episodic increases in EMG tone of the chin and masseter muscles.

Sleep-related choking syndrome	Abrupt awakenings with a choking sensation or inability to breathe, and accompanied by fear and anxiety. No stridor.	Can give rise to insomnia or sleep fragmentation.	
Sleep-related laryngospasm	Acute breathlessness due to total or near-total cessation of airflow during sleep that may be due to vocal cord spasm or tracheal swelling.	Sudden awakening accompanied by inspiratory stridor, temporary hoarseness and cyanosis.	
Sleep-related leg cramp	Sleep disturbance due to painful spasms or tightening of the muscles of the calf or foot.	Frequent leg cramps can result in insomnia or EDS.	Awakening that coincides with non-periodic bursts of high frequency EMG activity in the gastrocnemius muscle.
Sleep-related neurogenic tachypnea	Sustained tachypnea that develops during sleep.	May lead to sleep fragmentation and EDS.	
Sleep-related painful erection	Painful penile erections without apparent penile	Sleep-maintenance insomnia.	Events occur during REM sleep.

	disorder.		
Sleep start	Sudden muscle contraction of part or all of the body that occurs at sleep onset. Usually involves the legs, but can also affect the arms and head.	Can involve (a) a single, brief body jerk accompanied by a sensation of "falling"; (b) flashes of light or vivid imagery; (c) loud sound; or (d) somesthetic [floating] sensation.	Arousal or awakening from drowsiness or N1 sleep accompanied by brief EMG potentials.
Sleep talking	Vocalization during sleep.	No apparent clinical or psychological consequences.	Occurs in all sleep stages.
Snoring	Production of sound during sleep due to vibration of the UA structures.	Not associated with arousals, O_2 desaturation, apneas-hypopneas, hypoventilation or significant cardiac arrhythmias.	Snoring is often loudest during stage N3 sleep and diminishes during REM sleep.
Spinal cord disease		Insomnia and SRBD (especially in persons with quadriplegia).	

Stimulant-dependent sleep disorder	Sleep disturbance related to the use or discontinuation of stimulant medications.	Insomnia or EDS.	
Stroke		Insomnia, EDS and altered dreams. Increased risk of OSA and CSA/CSR.	
Subwakefulness syndrome	Subjective sensation of constant EDS without objective evidence of sleepiness.	No history of frequent napping.	Normal PSG and MSLT findings.
Sudden cardiac death	Peak from 6 AM to 12 PM and nadir from 12 AM to 6 AM in the general population.		
Sudden unexplained nocturnal death syndrome	Sudden death occurring during sleep without any apparent cause. Mostly affects healthy adult Southeast Asian males	Victims have been described to display moaning, screaming, violent motor activity or labored breathing for a few minutes prior to	

	between the ages of 25-44 years.	death.	
Terrifying hypnagogic hallucinations	Nightmares occurring at sleep onset. Sudden awakening is accompanied by intense fear, full alertness and vivid dream recall.		
Toxin-induced sleep disorder	Chronic exposure to toxins (heavy metals or chemicals).	Insomnia or EDS due to CNS excitation or depression, respectively.	

Pharmacology of sleep

Medications can be sedating ($\downarrow$ SOL, $\uparrow$ SE, $\downarrow$ WASO and $\uparrow$ TST [*high sleep input pattern*]) or alerting ($\uparrow$ SOL, $\downarrow$ SE, $\downarrow$ TST and $\uparrow$ WASO [*low sleep input pattern*]), or both, as a direct action, adverse reaction or withdrawal effect.

	Description
Antidepressants	PSG generally shows $\uparrow$ N3, $\uparrow$ REM SL and $\downarrow$ R (there are many exceptions to this pattern). Sudden discontinuation can cause REM sleep rebound. SSRIs can cause abnormal slow eye movements during NREM sleep (so called "Prozac eyes"). Some SSRIs are sedating (fluvoxamine and paroxetine) whereas others are alerting (citalopram and fluoxetine). Trazodone, a serotonin antagonist and reuptake inhibitor, is sedating. Sedating TCAs include amitriptyline, doxepin, imipramine and trimipramine, while alerting TCAs include protriptyline. Antidepressants, except for bupropion, can induce or worsen RLS or PLMD. SSRIs can induce RBD.
Hypnotic agents	Barbiturates, BZ receptor agonists and chloral hydrate act via the GABA receptor complex. They are sedating (high sleep input pattern). BZ receptor agonists also decrease N3 and REM sleep. Eszopiclone, zaleplon and zolpidem have minimal effects on N3 and REM sleep. Rebound insomnia following BZ discontinuation is more severe with short-acting compared to longer-acting agents. BZ can increase both spindle (12-14 Hz) and "pseudo-spindle" (14-18 Hz) density.
Sodium oxybate	A CNS depressant that acts via GABA-B and GHB receptors. Indicated for EDS/cataplexy in narcolepsy. FDA class III drug. Pregnancy category B. No significant tolerance, withdrawal or rebound effects.

Overdose may lead to coma and death. PSG shows ↓ N3.

Stimulants	Beneficial effects include (a) ↓ sleepiness and fatigue, (b) ↑ alertness, and (c) enhanced daytime performance and memory (improved reaction time). Adverse effects include increase in HR, BP and temperature; anxiety; headaches; and palpitations. High-dose regular use of *caffeine* can lead to tolerance and withdrawal symptoms. *Amphetamines* should be avoided in persons with severe underlying heart disease, cardiac arrhythmias or hypertension. High abuse potential. Adverse effects include tachyarrhythmias, chest pain, psychosis and anorexia/weight loss. *Modafinil and armodafinil* are indicated for EDS secondary to narcolepsy and SWD. It is also used for residual sleepiness in persons with OSA who are being treated with PAP therapy. Less potent than amphetamines. modafinil/armodafinil are also less likely to change sleep architecture, cause rebound insomnia, or lead to abuse. Stimulants are alerting (low sleep input pattern, ↑ N3 and ↑ R). Withdrawal can give rise to EDS (↑ SOL and ↑ TST) and ↑ R (REM sleep rebound).
Antipsychotics	Generally sedating (high sleep input pattern) and ↑ R. Acts by blocking wake-active neurotransmitter receptors (acetylcholine, dopamine, histamine, norepinephrine and serotonin).
Opioids	Generally sedating (high sleep input pattern) at high doses. May promote wakefulness at low doses. PSG features during opioid use include ↓ N3 and ↑ R. Insomnia and nightmares can develop during opioid discontinuation. May give rise to or worsen OSA, CSA, hypoventilation and Biot's respiration, but can improve symptoms of RLS.
Anticonvulsants	Generally sedating. Can either ↓ N3 sleep (gabapentin and tiagabine) or ↑ N3 sleep (lamotrigine).

Nicotine	Stimulates basal forebrain cholinergic neurons. Low sleep input pattern.
Drugs of abuse	*Cocaine*: ↓ TST and ↓ R with acute use; ↓ SOL, ↑ TST and ↑ R (occasionally SOREMPs) during acute withdrawal. *Heroin*: ↓ TST, ↓ N3 and ↓ R. *Marijuana*: acute use at low doses (sedating, ↑ TST, ↑ N3 and slight ↓ R), acute use at high doses (hallucinatory, ↓ N3 and ↓ R) and withdrawal (↑ SOL, ↓ TST and ↑ R). *Ecstasy*: ↓ TST and ↓ R with acute use.
Alcohol	Facilitates GABA and inhibits glutamate. Alcohol has a biphasic effect on sleep and waking (stimulating at low doses and on the rising phase of alcohol levels; and sedating at high doses and on the falling phase of alcohol levels).

Changes in sleep due to common medications and substances

Commonly prescribed medications can give rise to a variety of sleep-related complaints.

	Agents
Common medications and substances that can cause insomnia	(a) *Alcohol* [withdrawal from]; (b) *anorectic agents*; (c) *antidepressants* [bupropion, fluoxetine, protriptyline and venlafaxine]; (d) *antihypertensives* [metoprolol and propanolol]; (e) *antiparkinsonian drugs* [levodopa (high doses)]; (f) *bronchodilators* (albuterol and theophylline); (g) *decongestants* [phenylpropanolamine and pseudoephedrine]; (h) *nicotine*; (i) *steroids* (prednisone); and (l) *stimulants* [caffeine, cocaine, dextroamphetamine, methamphetamine, methylphenidate and modafinil/armodafinil]
Common medications and substances that can cause sedation	(a) *Anticonvulsants* [carbamazepine, gabapentin, phenobarbital, phenytoin, tiagabine and valproic acid]; (b) *antidepressants* (amitriptyline, desipramine, doxepin, fluvoxamine, imipramine, lithium, mirtazapine, nefazodone, nortriptyline, paroxetine and trazodone]; (c) *antiemetics* [metoclopramide, ondansetron, phenothiazines and scopolamine]; (d) *antihistamines* [1st generation H1 agents, such as diphenhydramine]; (e) *antiparkinsonian drugs* [pramipexole and ropinirole]; (f) *antipsychotics* [chlorpromazine, clozapine, haloperidol, olanzapine and thioridazine]; (g) *barbiturates*; (h) *benzodiazepine receptor agonists*; (i) *chloral hydrate*]; (j) *gamma-hydroxybutyrate* (sodium oxybate); (k) *melatonin* and melatonin receptor agonists; (l) *muscle relaxants*; (m) *narcotic agents*; and (n) *neuroleptic agents*

Common medications that can cause or worsen RLS or PLMD	(a) Anticonvulsants [phenytoin]; (b) antidepressants [MAOI, SSRI, TCA, lithium, mirtazapine and venlafaxine]; (c) anti-emetics [metoclopramide and prochlorperazine]; (d) antihistamines [diphenhydramine]; and (e) antipsychotics [haloperidol and perphenazine]
Common medications that can cause or worsen RBD	(a) Alcohol [withdrawal]; (b) antidepressants [MAOI, SSRI, TCA and venlafaxine]; (c) barbiturates; and (d) caffeine
Common medications that can cause or worsen abnormal dreams or nightmares	(a) Alcohol (withdrawal); (b) amphetamines; (c) antidepressants [MAOI, SSRI and TCA]; (d) antipsychotics; (e) barbiturates; (f) benzodiazepines; (g) beta-blockers [propranolol]; (h) corticosteroids; (i) donepezil; (j) efavirenz; (k) levodopa; (l) mirtazapine; (m) naproxen; (n) opioids; and (o) reserpine

Changes in sleep architecture due to common medications and substances

Important medication- and substance-induced changes in sleep architecture are listed in the following table.

	Agents
Increase N3 sleep	(a) Alcohol [acute ingestion]; (b) antipsychotics (olanzapine, risperidone and quetiapine); (c) carbamazepine; (d) gabapentin; (e) gamma hydroxybutyrate; (f) lithium; (g) mirtazapine; (h) nefazodone; and (i) trazodone
Decrease N3 sleep	(a) Alcohol [withdrawal]; (b) antipsychotics [clozapine]; (c) barbiturates; (d) benzodiazepines; and (e) stimulants
Increase REM sleep	(a) Alcohol [withdrawal]; (b) bupropion; (c) nefazodone; (d) reserpine; and (e) withdrawal of REM-suppressants
Decrease REM sleep	(a) Alcohol [acute ingestion]; (b) antidepressants [MAOI, SSRI, TCA and venlafaxine]; (c) stimulants [amphetamines and methylphenidate]; (d) barbiturates; (e) benzodiazepines; (f) lithium; and (g) narcotic agents
Increase REM SL	(a) Antidepressants [MAOI, SSRI, TCA and venlafaxine]; and (b) stimulant agents [amphetamine]
Decrease REM SL	(a) Bupropion; and (b) withdrawal of REM-suppressants

Genes and sleep

Many physiologic processes and clinical disorders related to sleep are, at least in part, under genetic control.

	Description
Sleep architecture	Higher degree of concordance in MZ than DZ twins for TST, SE, SOL, arousals, % sleep stages, density of rapid eye movements, density of NREM spindles and power spectrum density.
Sleep deprivation	Mutations in *Bmal 1, Clock, Cryptochrome 1/2, NPAS2* and *prokineticin 2* are associated with decreased response to SD. Polymorphism in the adenosine A2a receptor gene influences sensitivity to caffeine's effect on sleep.
Circadian rhythm	Circadian rhythms are controlled by autoregulated transcription-translation positive and negative feedback loops involving clock-related proteins and other regulatory factors. Mammalian circadian genes consist of *B-mal1, Casein kinase 1 (CK1), Clock (clk), Cryptochrome (Cry1* and *Cry2), Period (per1, per2 and per3),* and *Timeless (tim).* Other genes may be involved. An individual's chronotype ("eveningness" or "morningness") may be determined, in part, by the *Clock* gene. Mutations in clock genes are associated with faster or slower cycles than normal clocks.
Advanced sleep phase syndrome (familial)	Autosomal dominant variant of the disorder with a serine to glycine mutation in the casein kinase I epsilon (CKIε) binding region of *hPer2* (*human Period 2*) that is localized near the telomere of chromosome 2q. This causes hypophosphorylation of the hPer2 protein by CKIε and

161

Condition	Description
Delayed sleep phase syndrome	A positive family history may be present in 40% of affected persons. An autosomal dominant pattern of transmission has been described in a family with DSPS. Polymorphisms in the circadian clock genes, hPer3, Clock, CkIε, and arylalkylamine N-acetyltransferase, have been reported. results in shortening of the transcription-translation feedback loop cycle duration.
Insomnia	Higher concordance in MZ than DZ twins for insomnia symptoms. Mutation in the gene coding for a GABA-A β3 subunit has been described.
Fatal familial insomnia	Autosomal dominant disease involving a single point mutation at codon 178 of the prion protein gene on chromosome 20. Severity of the disease is influenced by codon 129, which can either be (a) methionine homozygous (more severe and shorter duration of illness before death); or (b) methionine-valine heterozygous (milder disease).
Narcolepsy	Risk of developing narcolepsy is 10-40 X greater among 1st degree relatives than in the general population. Risk of having an affected child is about 1%. Low concordance (1 in 3) among MZ twins (suggesting environmental trigger factors). Associated with certain HLA, namely DR2 (particularly the subtype DR15) and DQ1 (particular DQ6 [DQB1*0602]). DQB1*0602, the most important allele, is present in about 90% of narcolepsy with cataplexy and 40-60% of narcolepsy without cataplexy. Most multiplex family cases (multiple members of the family having narcolepsy) are HLA DQB1*0602 positive. However, it is neither sensitive nor specific for narcolepsy (it is also prevalent in the general population [12-25%] and most persons positive for

HLA DQB1*0602 do *not* have narcolepsy). There is a positive correlation between DQB1*0602 allele frequency (copy number) and symptom severity. Decreased hypocretin levels (autosomal recessive mutation of hypocretin receptor-2 [Hcrt2] gene in canine model; absence of hypocretin, hypocretin receptors or hypocretin neurons; knockout mice for the precursor ligand of the hypocretin receptor in rodent model; and pre-pro-hypocretin gene mutation in a case of early onset narcolepsy in human models). Polymorphism near carnitine palmitoyltransferase 1B (CPT1B) and choline kinase beta (CHKB) (*note: levels of both are lower*) in narcolepsy with cataplexy in Japan. Associated with specific single nucleotide peptides on the T-cell receptor alpha (TCRα) locus (*note: TCR interacts with HLA DQB1*0602*).

Idiopathic hypersomnia	Some persons may have an autosomal dominant mode of transmission. Association with HLA-Cw2 in some familial cases.
Obstructive sleep apnea	↑ Prevalence in 1st degree relatives. Risk increases with number of affected family members. 35% of the variance in disease severity can be attributed to genetic factors (independent of BMI). About 20-40% of the variance in AHI can be attributed to obesity-related genes.
Snoring	Higher degree of concordance in MZ than DZ twins.
Congenital central alveolar hypoventilation syndrome	Many cases involve *de novo* mutations in the PHOX2B gene.
Parasomnias	Higher degree of concordance in MZ than DZ twins for sleepwalking, sleep terrors, sleep

	enuresis and idiopathic sleep paralysis. RBD associated with HLA-DQB1*05 and DQB1*06 in some patients. Sleepwalking associated with HLA DQB1*0501. Up to 50% of persons with sleep bruxism may have a positive family history. Increasing prevalence of sleep enuresis related to the number of affected parents.
Restless legs syndrome	Positive family history in 90% of persons with primary RLS and 10% of persons with secondary RLS. Autosomal dominant transmission with incomplete penetrance in up to 30-60% of primary RLS. Higher degree of concordance in MZ than DZ twins. Presence of numerous susceptibility loci (chromosomes 2p, 2q, 4q/17p, 6p, 9q, 12q, 14q, 15q and 20p).
Sudden unexplained nocturnal death syndrome	Unknown pathogenesis. Mutation in the SCN5A gene is present in some families.

Sleep-related violence

There are 3 subgroups of nocturnal violent activity, namely (a) self-inflicted injuries; (b) injury to others; and (c) both.

	Description
Sleep disorders associated with sleep-related violence	(a) Confusional arousals; (b) medication and substance use; (c) RBD; (d) sleep terrors; (e) sleep-related seizures; (f) sleepwalking; and (g) sun downing.
Predisposing factors	(a) Disturbances in wake/sleep schedules; (b) dysfunctional families; (c) male gender; (d) history of physical or sexual abuse; (e) stress; and (f) substance abuse [drugs or alcohol].
Differential diagnoses	(a) Dissociative and fugue states; (b) drug-related states; (c) intentional homicide; (d) malingering; (e) Munchausen by proxy; (f) trance states; and (g) volitional waking behavior.
Evaluation	(a) Extensive neurological, psychiatric or neuropsychological assessment; (b) PSG [may need full scalp EEG in suspected seizures]; (c) wake and sleep EEGs; (d) non-attended ambulatory EEG in home environment; and (e) video-telemetry or simple home video recordings.
Therapy	(a) Avoidance of known facilitating and triggering factors; (b) proper sleep/wake hygiene; (c) avoidance of SD; and (d) measures to avoid injury.

Driving safety and vehicular accidents

SD and sleep-related disorders are frequent causes of preventable vehicular accidents.

	Description
General	↑ Risk of car accidents (particularly severe crashes) in sleepy persons with OSA. Effective therapy of OSA decreases this risk.
Risk factors	Features of EDS-related car accidents include (a) driving at high speeds; (b) involve single vehicles; (c) more common between 2-8 AM or during mid-late afternoon; (d) involve off-road accidents; (e) result in injuries, hospitalization or death; (f) victims are often young men; (g) < 5 hours of sleep during the night prior to the accident, and increased time awake; and (h) prolonged driving duration. SD of > 21-24 hours results in impairment comparable to a blood alcohol level of 0.08-0.10% (considered legally intoxicated). Furthermore, there are additive effects of sleep disruption and alcohol use on performance impairments.
Clinical evaluation	Regularly ask about history of drowsy driving and sleepiness-related accidents or near-miss accidents. Regularly ask about snoring, witnessed apneas (and other features suggestive of OSA), or other sleep disorders. A history of near-miss accidents predicts future risk of car accidents. Many persons with OSA misperceive the severity of their sleepiness (i.e., poor correlation between subjective measures and objective tests of sleepiness).
Diagnosis	Subjective or objective tests of sleepiness, AHI, degree of O_2 desaturation and performance on

	driving simulation tests do not reliably predict the risk of car accidents in persons with OSA.
Therapy	Counsel regarding sleep hygiene, including obtaining an adequate amount of sleep. Consider a trial of sleep extension in persons who are habitually sleep deprived. Instruct to avoid driving whenever drowsy. Avoidance of hypnotic agents if driving is anticipated. PAP therapy is preferred treatment for OSA; oral devices are not recommended because of inability to objectively measure adherence; UA surgery is acceptable but must document treatment efficacy. Assess adherence to PAP therapy in persons with OSA. Consider MSLT and/or MWT when in doubt about degree of sleepiness; however, MSLT and MWT data alone are not consistently able to predict safety risk. Consider a trial of modafinil/armodafinil for objectively determined residual sleepiness despite PAP therapy in persons with OSA. Consider other causes of EDS (e.g., narcolepsy or insufficient sleep syndrome). Schedule periodic follow-up. Understand national, regional and local laws and regulations related to sleep disorders and driving safety. Consider reporting the patient with EDS due to OSA to appropriate authorities, especially if (a) history of severe car accidents related to unexplained or untreated EDS; (b) prompt therapy for OSA cannot be provided; (c) patient refuses, or is consistently non-adherent with, therapy for OSA; (d) patient fails to restrict driving until OSA has been adequately controlled; or (e) such situations are considered reportable based on local laws.

The early years

There are significant differences in sleep architecture and manifestations of sleep disorders between children and adults. Newborn sleep is *polyphasic* (i.e., occurring repetitively and randomly throughout the 24-hour day). *Monophasic* sleep (occurring once, generally at night) develops during early childhood (ages 3-5 years) when napping ceases. Daily duration of sleep decreases from newborn infants (70% of 24-hour day) to adults (25-35% of 24-hour day).

In the 1st 6 months of life, sleep is classified as active sleep (REM sleep-equivalent), quiet sleep (NREM sleep equivalent), intermediate sleep or transitional sleep. Classification of sleep in infants older than 6 months of age is similar to that of adults (i.e., NREM or REM sleep).

Initial sleep episode can either be active [REM] sleep (< 3 months of age) or quiet [NREM] sleep (> 3-4 months of age). Proportion of NREM-REM sleep is 50:50 in infants and 75:25 among adolescents and adults. Sleep as a percentage of TST is greatest during early childhood and declines with aging. Percentage of REM sleep also decreases with aging, from 50% of TST (infants) to 25% of TST (adolescents and adults). NREM-REM cycle length (ultradian sleep rhythm) is ≈ 50-60 minutes during infancy and increases to ≈ 90-120 minutes in adults.

There is wide variability in optimal amount of sleep among children. TST gradually decreases throughout childhood from 16-19 hours each day in neonates (newborn-2 months) to 7-9 hours among adolescents (14-18 yrs). Decrease in sleep duration across early childhood is due mostly to reduction in daytime naps.

Sleep stages in the first 6 months of age

Sleep consists of 4 stages in the first 6 months of life, namely active, quiet, intermediate and transitional sleep.

	Description
Active sleep	First behavioral sleep state to appear. This is the predominant sleep state in the newborn period. Key features are body and facial twitches and jerks, variable muscle tone, rapid eye movements, and irregular respiration and HR. EEG shows a low-voltage pattern.
Quiet sleep	Becomes the predominant sleep state by 3 months of age. Key features are minimal or no body movements and regular respiration and HR. EEG shows high-voltage, slow-wave activity. Trace' alternant EEG pattern is present in the newborn and disappears by 1 month of age.
Intermediate sleep	Does not fully meet criteria for either active or quiet sleep.
Transitional sleep	Occurs in the transition between active, quiet and intermediate sleep.

Sleep stages after 6 months of age

Sleep is differentiated into 4 stages after 6 months of age (as listed below).

	EEG	EOG	EMG	Other features
Stage NREM 1	Desynchronized (low voltage, mixed frequency) activity	Absence of rapid eye movements; slow eye movements may be present	Low muscle tone	Regular respiration and HR; periodic breathing may be seen
Stage NREM 2	Rhythmic activity (e.g., sleep spindles and K-complexes)	Absence of eye movements	Low muscle tone	Regular respiration and HR
Stage NREM 3	High voltage, slow (< 4 Hz) frequency activity	Absence of eye movements	Low muscle tone	Regular respiration and HR
Stage REM	Desynchronized (low voltage, mixed frequency) activity	Episodic rapid eye movements (during phasic REM sleep)	Muscle atonia	Irregular respiration and HR

Developmental milestones in sleep architecture

Ages at which specific EEG features and sleep stages first appear are listed. Significant individual differences are present.

	First appearance
1-2 months	Sleep spindles
3 months	Delta waves
3-4 months	Dominant posterior alpha rhythm
4-6 months	K complexes
6 months	Distinct EEG features that allow differentiation among N1, N2 and N3 sleep
3-12 months	Hypnagogic hypersynchrony

Developmental milestones in sleep patterns

There is great individual variability in the ages during which developmental milestones in sleep patterns occur. Therefore, a specific sleep behavior in a child may be considered "normal-for-age" or "problematic" depending on physiological maturity, cultural perceptions and parental expectations. The following are the typical ages at which specific sleep-related behaviors commonly first develop.

	Developmental milestones
6 weeks	Longest sleep period occurring at night
2-3 months	Falling asleep on their own at bedtime (settling)
2-3 months	Falling back asleep on their own (self-soothing)
3-6 months	Nocturnal sleep consolidation (ability to sleep through the night)
3-6 years	Cessation of daytime napping

Developmental milestones in sleep-wake control

The SCN is functional *in utero.* Irregular sleep-wake rhythms are present immediately after birth.

	Developmental milestones
1 month	24-hr core body temperature rhythm develops
3 months	24-hr cycling of endogenous melatonin and cortisol production starts
2-4 months	Regular sleep-wake rhythms develop
4-5 months	Entrainment is present
6-12 years	Endogenous circadian sleep phase preference (e.g., eveningness vs. morningness) develops
12-18 years	Development of sleep phase delay

Childhood sleep disorders

Childhood sleep disorders often present differently from their adult counterparts.

	Description
Hypersomnia	EDS should be considered in any child > 5 years of age who (a) continues to nap during the day, especially if unplanned; (b) sleeps $\geq$ 2 hours more on weekends than on weekdays ("weekend oversleep"); (c) falls asleep at inappropriate times and situations; or (d) has behavioral problems (inattentiveness, irritability, hyperactivity or impulsiveness). Other common features include cognitive problems or academic difficulties, changes in mood (depression or anxiety), fatigue and lethargy.
Insomnia	Causes include (a) adjustment sleep disorder [e.g., acute stress or change in bedroom environment]; (b) bedtime resistance; (c) colic [sustained episodes of crying (> 3 hours), irritability or fussing, with no apparent reason]; (d) food allergy; (e) limit-setting sleep disorder [repetitive refusal by a child to go to sleep at an appropriate time due to inadequate enforcement of bedtimes by the caregiver]; (f) nighttime fears; (g) psychophysiologic insomnia; (h) separation anxiety; and (i) sleep-onset association disorder [inability to fall asleep, or return to sleep after an awakening, without the presence of certain desired but inappropriate, objects or parental intervention].
Snoring	May be associated with EDS, behavioral and cognitive problems (attention, language, memory

and executive function), and mood disorders.

Apnea of prematurity	Obstructive or central apneas/hypopneas in infants < 37 weeks of gestation. May also present with periodic breathing. Respiratory events may be associated with bradycardia, hypoxemia or need for caregiver intervention.
Infant sleep apnea	Obstructive or central apneas/hypopneas in infants > 37 weeks of gestation. Central events are more common than obstructive events. Respiratory events can be associated with hypoxemia, brady-tachycardia, cyanosis and arousals.
Apparent life-threatening event	Clinical features include: (a) apnea, (b) change in color or tone (limpness) and (c) choking or gagging. Responds to stimulation or resuscitation.
Sudden infant death syndrome	Sudden unexpected death of an infant < 1 year of age that remains unexplained after a thorough post-mortem assessment, including review of medical history, scene of death investigation and autopsy.
Childhood obstructive sleep apnea	Clinical features include EDS, snoring, witnessed apneas, unusual sleep posture [e.g., hyperextended neck], labored or paradoxical breathing and thoracic retractions, cognitive or behavioral difficulties, and mood changes. PSG features consist of pauses in breathing or reduction in airflow by greater than 30-50% compared to baseline, lasting ≥ 2 normal respiratory cycles; ≥ *1 scoreable respiratory event per hour*. Obstructive hypoventilation consists of prolonged periods of persistent partial UA obstruction with hypercapnia ± O_2 desaturation. Adenotonsillectomy is the treatment of choice for most children with OSA but incomplete

--	resolution of OSA following adenotonsillectomy is common. Consider CPAP if UA surgery is not indicated, contraindicated or ineffective (failed adenotonsillectomy).
Restless legs syndrome	Definite diagnosis (ages 2-12 years) requires all adult criteria for RLS _and_ description of leg discomfort in the child's own words _or_ ≥ 2 of the following (sleep disturbance; biological parent or sibling with definite RLS; or PLMI index > 5 per hour during PSG).

Behavioral treatment of childhood sleep disturbance

Behavioral therapy is highly effective for many causes of childhood sleep disturbance.

	Description
General measures	Parental education. Placing a child to bed while drowsy but still awake (to teach a child to fall asleep independently) beginning at 2-3 months of age. Transitioning the infant to the final sleep environment (e.g., crib in infant's room) by 3 months of age. Discontinuation of nighttime feedings in children ≥ 6 months of age.
Bedtime management	Maintenance of consistent bedtimes. Age-appropriate bedtime. Establishment of optimal sleep-friendly bedroom environment. Appropriate use of transitional objects (e.g., doll or blanket) for sleep-onset association disorder. Consistent and predictable parental enforcement of bedtimes for limit setting sleep disorder.
Positive bedtime routines	Establishing consistent and relaxing pre-bedtime activities.
Faded bedtime	Bedtime is progressively delayed (e.g., by 30 minutes) until the child is able to fall asleep rapidly. Subsequent bedtimes are then advanced or delayed depending on SOL until the desired bedtime is reached.
Scheduled awakening	The child is awakened by the parent slightly before the usual spontaneous time of awakening, reassured, and then allowed to return to sleep. Frequency of scheduled awakenings is

	progressively decreased until they are discontinued completely once the child is able to sleep through the night.
Extinction techniques	Three general types, namely fast approach, gradual approach or extinction with parental presence. *Fast approach* (absolute extinction) involves putting the child in bed, leaving the child alone in the room, and ignoring inappropriate behavior and unreasonable demands until the next morning. *Gradual approach* (graduated extinction) differs from the fast approach in that parents are allowed to respond to a child's inappropriate demands in a gradually decreasing fashion (i.e., longer duration between interventions or shorter periods of intervention) until parental intervention is finally stopped. *Extinction with parental presence* permits the parent to sleep in a separate bed in the child's bedroom but not to respond to any inappropriate behavior by the child.
Cognitive behavioral therapy	Sleep restriction, stimulus control and cognitive therapy as in adults.
Pharmacologic treatment	No hypnotic agent is currently approved by the US FDA for use in children. Neither the efficacy nor safety of melatonin has been established for children.

Aging

Sleep requirements do not decline with aging. Aging is associated with greater nocturnal sleep disturbance (prevalence of 50%), EDS and daytime napping. While some of the sleep disturbance can be attributed to normal aging itself (sleep homeostasis and circadian rhythms), most are due to comorbid medical (menopause or nocturia), neurological (dementia), psychiatric (depression) or primary sleep disorders; the adverse effects on sleep of medications used to treat them; and diminished arousal threshold and greater sensitivity to environmental disturbances. Older women are better able to maintain satisfactory sleep with aging compared to older men. Disturbed sleep is a common reason for institutional placement for aging adults. Other consequences of disturbed sleep among older adults are impairments in attention, memory, response time and performance; ↑ risk of falls; ↑ use of healthcare resources; and, possibly, ↓ survival.

What stays the same	What increases	What decreases
Sleep requirements	(a) Nocturnal sleep disturbance; (b) EDS; (c) frequency of napping; (d) tolerance to SD; and (e) prevalence of insomnia, OSA, CSA, RLS, PLMD, RBD, ASPD, SWD and JL	(a) N3 sleep; (b) melatonin secretion; (c) amplitude of circadian sleep-wake rhythms; (d) homeostatic sleep drive; (e) arousal threshold; (f) GH secretion during sleep; and (g) tolerance to shift work and JL

Physiologic changes with aging

Aging is associated with changes in several physiologic processes related to sleep and wakefulness.

	Description
Circadian and homeostatic systems	↓ Melatonin secretion, ↓ amplitude of circadian sleep-wake rhythms, phase advancement of circadian sleep-wake rhythms (starting at middle adulthood) and ↓ homeostatic sleep drive
Arousal threshold	↓ Arousal threshold and ↑ sensitivity to adverse environmental factors
Endocrine system	↓ GH secretion during sleep, and ↓ nighttime and daytime levels of testosterone
Thermoregulation	↑ CTmin, ↓ ability to lose heat to the periphery, ↓ responsiveness to thermal changes and ↓ circadian temperature rhythm amplitude
Sleep and sleep patterns	↓ Sleep quality, ↑ sleep disturbance, ↑ nighttime awakenings and ↑ daytime naps
Sleep architecture	↓ SE, ↑ SOL, ↑ WASO, ↓/= TST, ↑ N1, ↓ N3, ↓ REM SL and ↓/= R
Sleep disorders	↑ Prevalence of insomnia, OSA, CSA, RLS, PLMD, RBD and ASPS

Sleep disorders in the older adult

Older adults are at increased risk of developing insomnia and OSA.

	Description
Insomnia	Most common sleep complaint among older adults. More frequently involves sleep-maintenance insomnia. Risk factors include depression, disability, poor health, medical disorders, respiratory symptoms, sedative use, bereavement, widowhood and other concurrent primary sleep disorders. Rarely due exclusively to aging itself.
Obstructive sleep apnea	Compared to younger adults, older adults generally have decreased frequency and severity of OSA-related EDS; milder nocturnal O_2 desaturation; less risk of cardiopulmonary diseases; less association with obesity, snoring, witnessed apneas, HTN and cognitive dysfunction; and similar PAP adherence rates.
Nocturia	May develop due to ↓ urinary bladder capacity, ↓ urinary concentrating ability, prostatic enlargement (in men), detrussor overactivity or comorbid OSA (weak correlation with AHI).

Sleep in women

Women generally have ↑ subjective complaints of insufficient or nonrestorative sleep as well as ↑ need for sleep compared to men. However, they typically have better objective parameters of sleep (↑ SE, ↑ TST and ↑ N3) during PSG than men. There is a higher prevalence of insomnia, RLS and dissatisfaction with sleep compared to men.

	Description
Obstructive sleep apnea	OSA is less common in pre-menopausal women than in men. Risk of OSA increases in women during menopause. Women are generally more symptomatic at comparable AHIs than men. Differences in clinical presentation (compared to men) include ↓ snoring, ↓ witnessed apneas, ↑ insomnia, ↑ EDS and fatigue, ↓ functional status, ↑ morning headaches and ↑ mood disturbance. Differences in PSG features (compared to men) are lower AHI (when matched for body weight), ↓ supine position dependency of respiratory events, ↓ O_2 desaturation and ↓ survival rates compared to men with similar AHIs.
Central sleep apnea	Less common in premenopausal women than in men.
Insomnia	Prevalence of insomnia is increased (a) during pre-menstrual (late luteal) and early menstrual phases, (b) during and after pregnancy, and (c) during peri/postmenopause.
Menstrual cycle	Sleep quality can deteriorate prior to and during the first several days of menstruation. Sleep-related complaints include insomnia and EDS, and can be caused by abdominal bloating and cramping, anxiety, breast tenderness, headaches or mood changes.

Oral contraceptive use	Increase in mean levels of melatonin. Increased body temperature during sleep. PSG features include ↑ N1, ↑N2, ↓/= N3 and ↓ REM SL.
Pregnancy	Sleep quality during pregnancy is worse during 1st trimester, improves during 2nd trimester, and worst during 3rd trimester. Common causes of sleep disturbance during pregnancy include anxiety, back pain, breast tenderness, dyspnea, fetal movements, heartburn and GER, leg cramps, nausea and vomiting (morning sickness), nocturia (worse during 1st and 3rd trimesters), RLS, and snoring or OSA. PSG features consist of ↓ SE, ↑ WASO, ↑ TST (decreases by late pregnancy), ↑ N1, ↑ N2, ↓/= N3 and ↓ R (during late pregnancy). Associated with ↑ risk of snoring, OSA, RLS/PLMD, nocturnal leg cramps and EDS.
Labor and delivery	Shorter TST (< 6 hrs) prior to labor and delivery is associated with longer labor and increased likelihood of cesarean delivery compared to longer nighttime sleep duration (> 7 hrs).
Postpartum period	EDS, cognitive impairment, changes in mood and ↑ frequency of napping may be seen. PSG features are ↓ SE, ↓ TST, ↑ WASO, ↓ N1, ↓ N2, ↑ N3, and no change in R and REM SL.
Menopause and post-menopause	Common complaints include hot flashes, night sweats, insomnia, mood changes, fatigue and EDS. Increased prevalence of OSA.
Aging	Sleep in healthy older women (compared to older men) is characterized by ↑ frequency of insomnia, poorer sleep quality, ↑ need for daytime naps, ↑ use of sedative-hypnotic agents and less changes in sleep architecture (no significant ↓ in N3).

Hormone replacement therapy	Therapy with oral synthetic estrogens and progesterone can have beneficial effects on sleep, including improvement in sleep quality, and ↓ prevalence of OSA, insomnia and hot flashes. PSG effects are ↑ SE, ↓ SOL, ↑ TST, ↓ WASO and ↑ N3.

Appendix

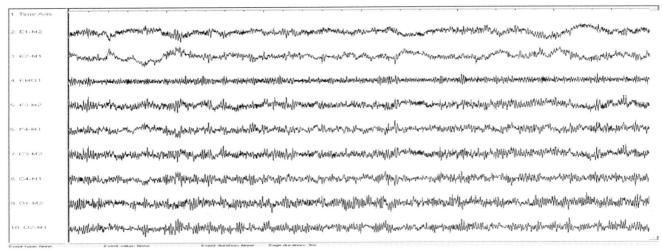

Stage W

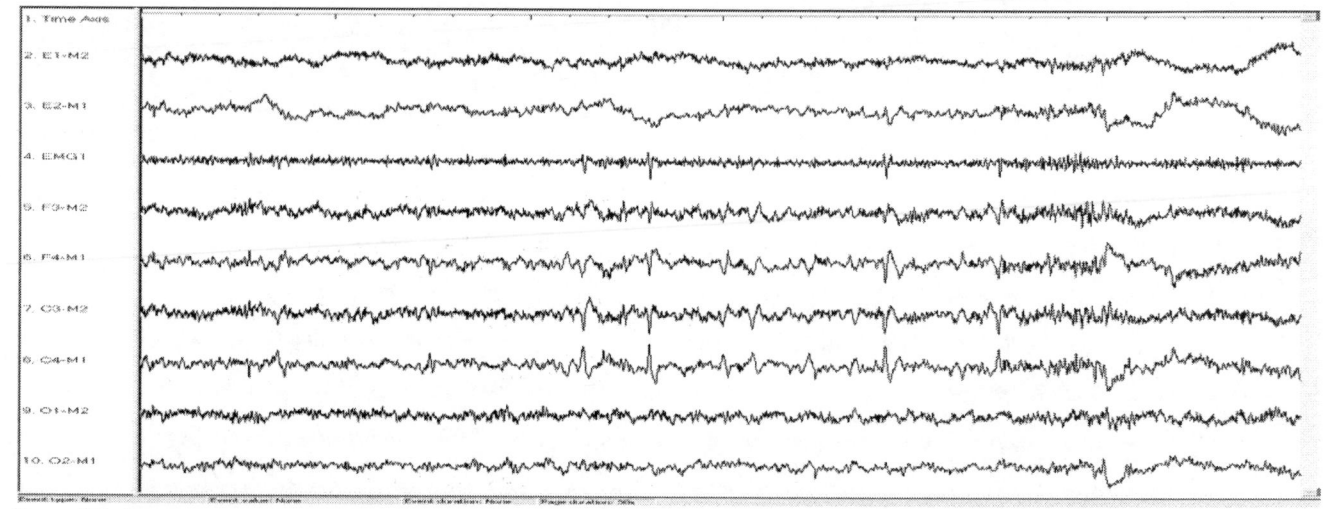

Stage N1 sleep

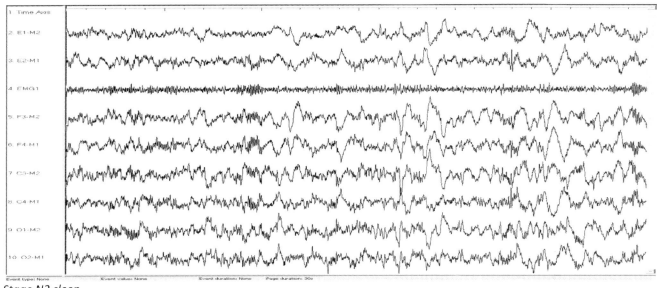

Stage N2 sleep

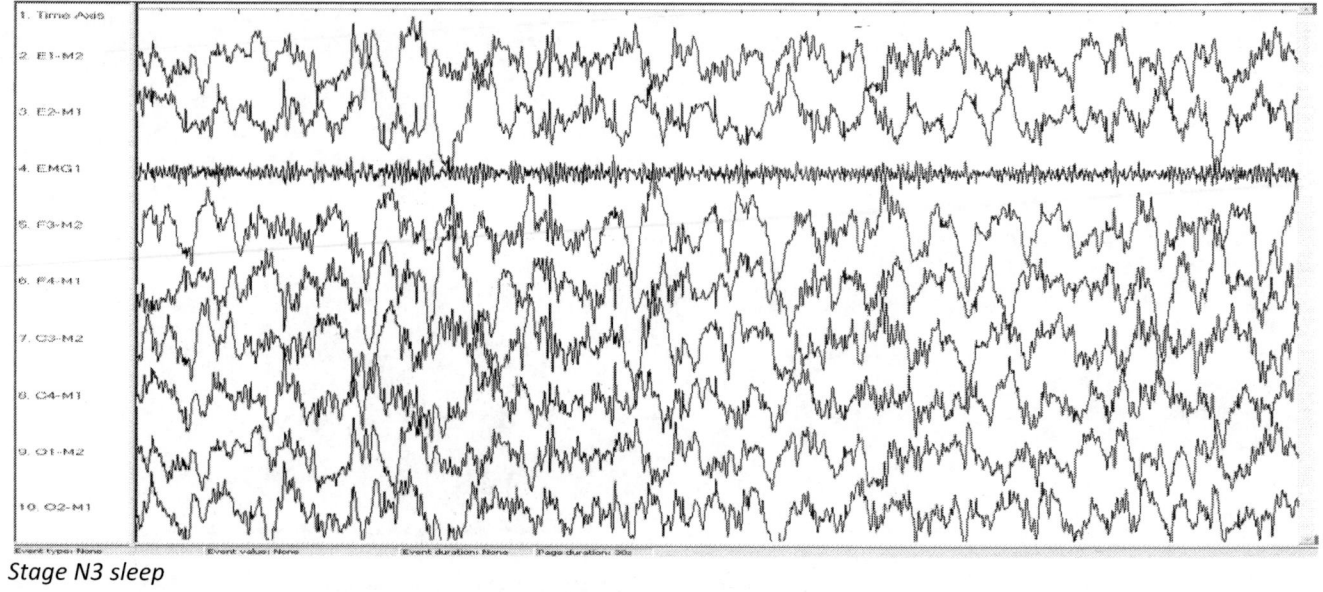

Stage N3 sleep

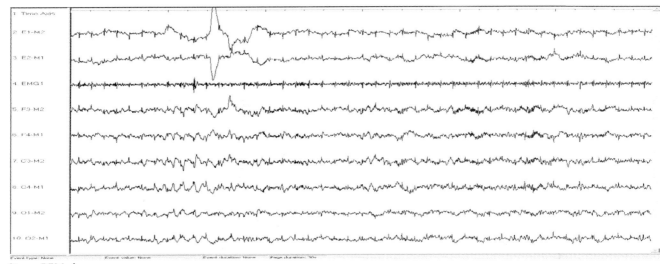

Stage REM sleep

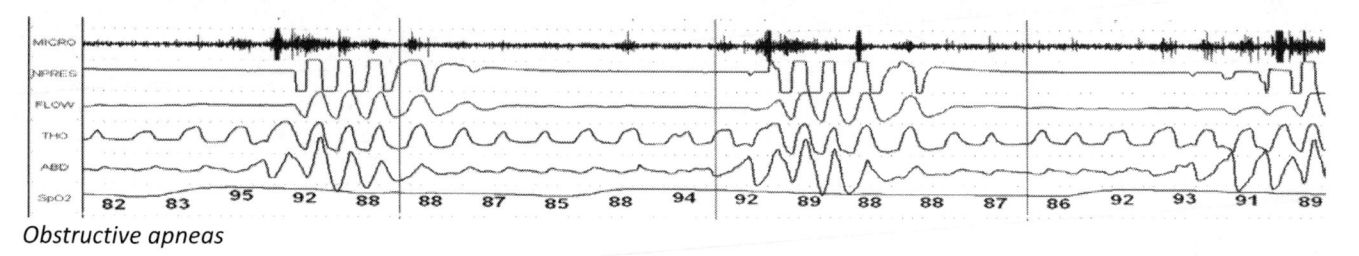

Obstructive apneas

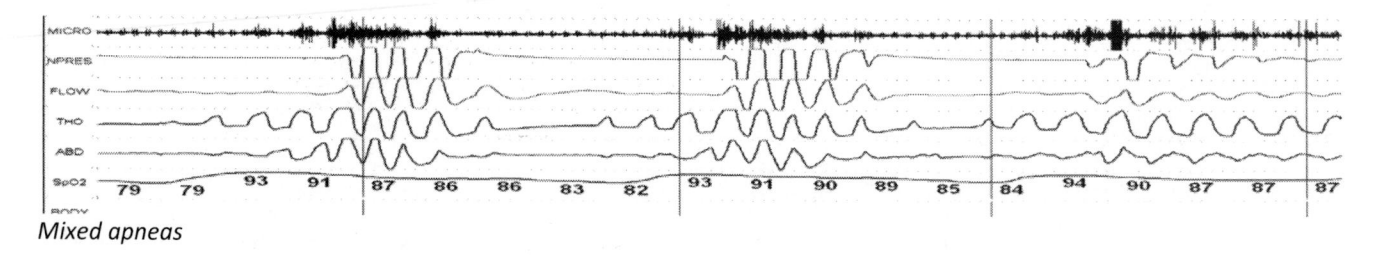

Mixed apneas

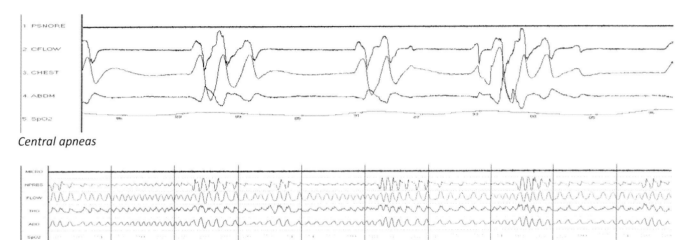

Central apneas

Hypopneas

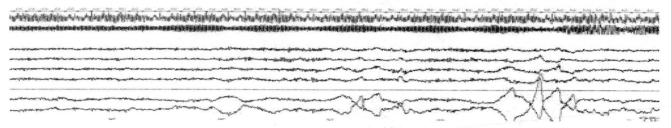

Bruxism

60 Hz artifact

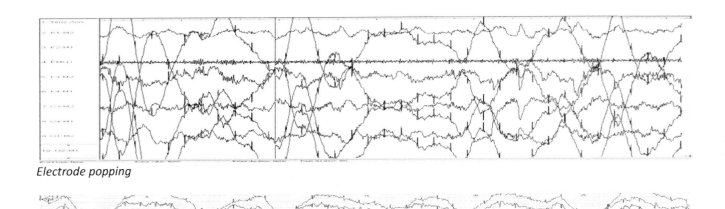

Electrode popping

Sweat artifact

Major references

1. American Academy of Sleep Medicine. The International Classification of Sleep Disorders, Second Edition: Diagnostic and Coding Manual. American Academy of Sleep Medicine. 2005.
2. Iber C, Ancoli-Israel S, Chesson A, and Quan SF for the American Academy of Sleep Medicine. The AASM Manual for the Scoring of Sleep and Associated Event Rules: Terminology and Technical Specifications, 1st Ed: Westchester, Illinois: American Academy of Sleep Medicine, 2007.
3. Lee-Chiong T. Best of Sleep Medicine 2010. Createspace Press, 2010.
4. Lee-Chiong T. Best of Sleep Medicine 2011. Createspace Press, 2011.
5. Lee-Chiong T. Sleep Medicine: Essentials and Review. Oxford University Press, 2008.
6. Lee-Chiong TL (Ed). Sleep: A Comprehensive Handbook. John Wiley & Sons, Hoboken, New Jersey, 2006.
7. Sleep Research Society. SRS Basics of Sleep Guide. Sleep Research Society. 2009.

Disclaimer

No individual is perfect – and certainly *not* this author. Every effort has been made to verify the accuracy of the facts in this book. Any errors that were missed will be incorporated in future editions. In the meantime, kindly accept my sincere apology if any correction has been overlooked or if any concept has not been satisfactorily presented.

Index

Important numbers

Sleep laboratory

_____
_____
_____

Sleep medicine clinic

_____
_____
_____

Medical center

_____
_____

Emergency department

_____

Pharmacy _____

Security _____

Medical director

_____

Sleep center director

_____

Sleep laboratory manager

_____

Sleep physician/s

_____
_____
_____
_____
_____
_____

Made in the USA
San Bernardino, CA
30 August 2016

37882392R00116